Building Strength and Muscle After 50

Chad Landers

HUMAN KINETICS

Library of Congress Cataloging-in-Publication Data

Library of Congress Cataloging-in-Publication information is available. LCCN 2025029912 (print).

ISBN: 978-1-7182-2388-2 (print)

Acquisitions Editors: Korey Van Wyk and Michelle Earle
Senior Developmental Editor: Cynthia McEntire
Managing Editor: Kevin Matz
Copyeditor: Laura Whittemore/Kingbird Editorial
Graphic Designer: Denise Lowry
Cover Designer: Keri Evans
Cover Design Specialist: Susan Rothermel Allen
Photograph (cover): Michael Yates
Photographs (interior): Michael Yates/© Human Kinetics, unless otherwise noted
Photo Production Specialist: Amy M. Rose
Photo Production Manager: Jason Allen
Senior Art Manager: Kelly Hendren
Illustrations: © Human Kinetics
Printer: Sheridan Books

We thank PUSH Private Fitness in Toluca Lake, California, for assistance in providing the location for the photo shoot for this book.

Human Kinetics books are available at special discounts for bulk purchase. Special editions or book excerpts can also be created to specification. For details, contact the Special Sales Manager at Human Kinetics.

Printed in the United States of America   10 9 8 7 6 5 4 3 2 1

The paper in this book is certified under a sustainable forestry program.

Human Kinetics
1607 N. Market Street
Champaign, IL 61820
USA

United States and International
Website: **US.HumanKinetics.com**
Email: info@hkusa.com
Phone: 1-800-747-4457

Human Kinetics' authorized representative for product safety in the EU is Mare Nostrum Group B.V., Mauritskade 21D, 1091 GC Amsterdam, The Netherlands.
Email: gpsr@mare-nostrum.co.uk

E9239

CONTENTS

FOREWORD

Duff McKagan

I came across Chad sometime in the early 2000s. My life was full, with a wife and two little girls, and my life in music was going into full-throttle mode with touring and all that comes with that. I'd been sober, off booze and drugs, for about nine years when we met, and he helped me immensely with not only fitness (he's real good at that) but also with centering the whole. Mind. Body. Spirit.

I don't really think about age or aging—rather, my thing is to try to get better and better and break new personal bests—but Chad, while for sure helping with all this physical furtherment, is much more about me being able to handle my own body weight and balance and posture. These are indeed the things we need for comfort in our path to longevity. Strength, grace, and a sense of center.

My touring these days is at an all-time high. The shows we play can be three-and-a-half hours long, and we go out for months and months at a time. The gigs are one thing, but the travel and time changes and diet are all elements of what one needs to train for. Crossing paths with Chad has had long-lasting effects on how I approach taking care of myself at all times.

Chad has a ton of experience training all ages and body types. The knowledge he shares in this book about physical fitness is indeed a mountainous fountain of insight. Chad Landers is the real deal, and I am proud to be one small part of his story.

"I want to be a muscle man!" Some kids say astronaut, some say firefighter, police officer, or doctor . . . not me. When asked what I wanted to be when I grew up, my reply was always the same: "I want to be a muscle man!" This was the early 1970s, when Arnold Schwarzenegger won most of his Mr. Olympia titles, so my guess is that I saw him on a talk show (television was my babysitter, as it was for a lot of Gen-X latchkey kids) and was enamored with his gargantuan physique.

I requested my first set of dumbbells for my ninth birthday, which my uncle, Glenn, was happy to provide, and I've been lifting weights more or less ever since. Serious training didn't really begin until seventh grade when I started playing organized tackle football in junior high. I was your typical 98-pound weakling and needed to get MUCH stronger to improve my athleticism and, more importantly, for my own survival.

So, I saved my lawn mowing and farm chores money until I had enough to buy an Earl Campbell model weight bench from Sears. (For those who don't remember, Earl Campbell was a massive football player for the Houston Oilers franchise in the '70s.) For years I toiled in the basement of our farmhouse in rural Illinois. I ordered my first weight training book, Robert Kennedy's *Hardcore Bodybuilding: The Blood, Sweat and Tears of Pumping Iron*, and became enthralled by the physiques contained within, which further amplified my pursuit of building big muscles. Of course, at that time I had no clue that those physiques came by way of performance-enhancing drugs. I just knew they looked like superheroes, and that's how I wanted to look.

In high school, I got my first taste of the commercial gym experience while training at a hole-in-the-wall powerlifting gym in Galesburg, Illinois, called Brad's Gym. Football players from several area high schools would congregate there to train because Brad's was the only hardcore training gym in the county. I loved being a part of gym culture—everyone, even bitter football rivals, worked hard and cheered each other on to new personal records. This was the mid-1980s, long before the Internet or social media or camera phones existed. You went to the gym to train, not to create content for some group of nebulous "followers." It was glorious.

After high school, when my football playing days were over, I still pursued the iron—this time more driven to attract girls than to further my athletic pursuits. My freshman year at the University of Illinois was to be the major turning point in my life. While on campus I discovered that I could actually major in something called *kinesiology*, or the study of human movement. I quickly changed from a biology major to a "kines" major and continued my quest to become a muscle man.

When I switched majors, I honestly had no idea how I would make a living with a degree in kinesiology. I just knew it combined sciences like biology, anatomy, and physiology with my love of sports and weight training. I would find a way to earn a paycheck later. Fortunately, while still in school, I began training at an off-campus gym in Urbana called the Body Firm. It was not a hardcore, dank type of gym like Brad's, but rather it was bright, energetic, and fun!

I soon discovered that a fellow kines student who was an Urbana local worked part time at the Body Firm. I asked him if he could get me an interview, and before long, I had my first job at a gym. I would work there for three years, co-managing the place for the last two. It was a wonderful experience, and I cherish those memories of the gym culture we had at "the Firm." Thanks to social media, I've been able to stay in contact with dozens of people from that era.

In 1992, I decided to leave Illinois in hopes of pursuing a more lucrative career in fitness in a larger city. I ended up moving to Las Vegas because I had a free place to stay with my mom and stepdad. I endured Vegas for 10 months, working here and there, first in a shoe store, then at a luxury gym called the Las Vegas Sporting House, eventually ending up in the health spa at Bally's casino. I hated living in Vegas. But my job in the health spa put me in contact with people from all over the country, and I received many job offers from various spa patrons.

I ultimately took a job in Los Angeles as a personal trainer with a new training studio called IFC in 1993. I had trained people informally, but this would be the first time I'd have to make a living through personal training. Although I only spent two years at IFC before going out on my own, I met many clients who I would train for years to come—including my wife, Karen.

For the next eight years I would train my clients as an independent trainer at a Gold's Gym in North Hollywood. Gold's had neither the gritty charisma of Brad's Gym nor the friendly camaraderie of the Body Firm. Gold's was a means to an end. At the end of 2002, after years of searching for an appropriate space, I was finally able to open my gym, PUSH Private Fitness. I've been in the same location for nearly 23 years now.

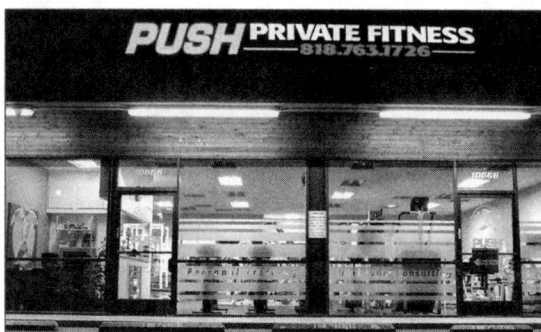

I share my history with you to show that I've seen it all and done it all over the past 32+ years as a personal trainer. I've worked in every type of gym and seen dozens of fitness and health fads come and go. I've trained children, the elderly, competitive athletes, celebrities, and more. I know what works, and I know how to simplify the pursuit of strength to make it both enjoyable and repeatable. And those things are what make the difference in whether you achieve your goals or give up.

You must enjoy what you're doing (or at a minimum, enjoy the results of your training) so that you can be consistent enough to do it long term. Under the best circumstances, results are slow and take time. And after you achieve your goals, you'll still need to train to maintain your gains.

This book contains everything I've learned over more than 36 years in the fitness industry. It is a simple guide to incorporate training into the busiest schedule and will help anyone looking to build strength and muscle after 50 achieve the results they desire.

Happy training!

Many people made this book possible. I'm going to attempt to keep the focus tight and as directly tied to this book as possible. But know that this endeavor is the culmination of a career of more than three decades, so there are countless people who've nurtured, supported, inspired, and influenced me who will unfortunately go unnamed.

A huge debt of gratitude goes to those who raised me: my late grandmother, Frances Landers, whose unconditional love and support saved me on more than one occasion, and my late uncle, Glenn Landers, who gave me my first set of dumbbells on my ninth birthday. I miss you both every day.

I thank grade-school teacher Sharon Peterson, who instilled in me a love for creative writing, and fellow ROVA English teachers Judy Nolan, Jeanne Harland, Janet Mottaz, and Dan Renwick who taught me the power of words.

In 1989, Dan McCulley and Jim Maurer of the Body Firm in Urbana, Illinois, gave me my start in the gym business and showed me daily just how fun gym culture could be. Lance Fessler at IFC launched my career as a personal trainer in Los Angeles in 1993. Thank you.

I thank the PUSH Private Fitness family, especially the trainers who helped shape PUSH's empowering, inclusive vibe including Chris "Showerboy" Showerman, Mallory and Jimmy Hewell-Joseph, Tim Rivers, Jeff "Tree" Judd, Bobby Edner, and especially Victor Bayliss, my right-hand man for nearly two decades. I couldn't have done it without you.

Thank you to the many clients who entrusted me over the last three decades, some long before PUSH was in existence, especially long-term clients Barbara (RIP) and Ray Garmon (25 years each), Frances Kumashiro (29 years), and Donna Zimmerman (23 years and whose family and referrals made up over 50 percent of my schedule early in my career).

I thank the numerous actors and musicians I've worked with, especially Billy Zabka, Stephen Perkins, Corbin Bleu, Catherine Dent, Douglas Smith, Robbie Amell, Italia Ricci, Grey Damon, Camryn Grimes, Jack Falahee, and Jimmy D'Anda for their public support and vocal endorsements of me on this book's back cover and website materials, and especially to Duff McKagan, a true Renaissance man, stalwart friend, and sweaty bastard, for his unforgettable, heartfelt foreword.

The many fitness industry friends and colleagues who have inspired me are too numerous to mention individually, but I want to especially thank Jonathan Goodman, who gave me my first paid writing and paid speaking gigs; Martin Rooney and Bill Parisi, whose mentorship program in 2010 altered the trajectory of my career; Mark Fisher, Lee Boyce, and Nick Tumminello, the sources of countless referrals from back East; and Robert Linkul, Lavanya Krishnan, Dr. Mike T. Nelson, Sol Orwell, Andy Morgan, and Andrew Coates, some of my biggest behind-the-scenes supporters. Thanks also to Sean Hyson, Chad Waterbury, Charlie Weingroff, Lindsay Vastola, Lou Schuler, Mike Zimmerman, Tom Venuto,

Will Garcia, Stephen Alexander Ellis, Mike Howard, Tim Arndt, Scott Caulfield, Justin Kavanaugh, Kevin Dineen, Jeff Aker, and James Krieger.

I thank the Human Kinetics team: Korey Van Wyk (hat tip to Andrew Coates for the introduction), Michelle Earle, Cynthia McEntire, Kevin Matz, Jim Bowling, Alexis Koontz, Ellie Larson, and more. Your patience, polish, and professionalism elevated every page.

Photographer Michael Yates and Team PUSH Gen-X fitness models Olun Riley, Chris Showerman, and Sara Azari brought the exercises to life and are living proof of the power of strength training past 50.

I thank Angela Dufour, sports dietitian extraordinaire, whose expertise for chapter 3 rock-solidified this book.

For Karen Baker Landers—client-turned-wife, fearless critic, and eternal champion—no one is more responsible for my success than you! You never let me get away with giving less than my best. Thank you! I love you more than milk!

And a final thanks to my Gen-X brothers and sisters reading this book. I hope these pages pump you up as much as writing them did me. Get strong. Stay strong. Rock on.

When the sitcom *The Golden Girls* premiered in September 1985 (the start of my senior year in high school), the youngest cast member, Rue McClanahan, was 51 years old. Imagine, in 2025, casting J Lo (56), Jennifer Aniston (56), or Halle Berry (59) as Blanche. Impossible, right?

Or consider the film *Cocoon*, also from 1985. Costar Wilford Brimley (have you had your Quaker Oats today?) was only 50 years old at the time! Would anyone put Brad Pitt (62) or Tom Cruise (63) in that role today? I don't think so.

Then there are my current and former clients who were huge in the '80s and are *still* kicking ass today: Billy Zabka from *The Karate Kid* and *Cobra Kai*, drummer Stephen Perkins of Jane's Addiction and Porno for Pyros, and bassist Duff McKagan of Guns N' Roses all still thriving while filming and touring well into their 50s!

What enables today's quinquagenarians (yes, it's a real word!) to be so active, strong, and vibrant at an age when prior generations would have been happy sitting on the front porch in a rocking chair?

It may not be the youthful dip in the swimming pool filled with alien life force in *Cocoon*, but today's 50-somethings do have their own fountain of youth—strength training.

Although strength training has been around for well over a century, for most of that time it was considered more of a side show. Be it a vaudevillian strong man act or a male bodybuilding competition, strength training was considered the purview of freaks and egotists. And heaven forbid a woman touch a weight for fear of bulking up.

Even the fitness boom of the 1970s largely left out strength training. Jogging and aerobics were the popular exercises of the day, and books like Kenneth Cooper's *Aerobics* (1968) and *The New Aerobics* (1970) were selling millions of copies. And millions more running shoes were flying off the shelves by new companies called Nike and Brooks.

With the widespread availability of the VCR, 1982's *Jane Fonda's Workout* became the first nontheatrical home video release to top the sales chart. Indeed, fitness was booming, and cardio was king!

At first glance it all made perfect sense. Cardiovascular exercise strengthens the heart and lungs, and since heart disease had been the leading cause of death in the United States since 1950 (and still is), cardio was naturally thought to be the be-all and end-all of exercise, especially for older people.

Not to say that weight training wasn't gaining fans of its own. The physique that Arnold Schwarzenegger displayed in his charismatic turn in 1977's documentary *Pumping Iron* (along with his later action hero films and those of fellow pumped-up actors like Sylvester Stallone and Jean-Claude Van Damme) got lots of guys, me included, to start pumping iron ourselves. (Although women were still discouraged from their own muscular pursuits.)

Even most athletic coaches of the era thought weight training was a detriment to athletic development and would slow you down. "All show and no go" some would say.

But while strength training for sports was finally accepted and has been for decades, only recently has research shown how beneficial pumping iron is for older people too. While cardiovascular exercise is certainly important, we are now realizing that strength training confers a host of benefits that cardio doesn't.

Hopefully, if you've picked up this book, I'm preaching to the choir here. We 50-somethings were the first generation that actively started going to gyms and lifting weights en masse. And whether you've kept training since the '80s like I have, or you haven't set foot in the gym since the cassette tape era, you know that stronger is better than weaker.

But if it has been a long time since you've touched a weight, I understand you might have some reservations about jumping back into it. "Am I too old?" "What about my bum knee?" "I just don't think I have the time!"

Many of my clients initially had the same fears. I tell them two things: First, you're too old *not* to strength train. Second, strength never gets old. It's strength that helps avoid the midlife misery of pulling a muscle while sneezing or the horror of waking up with a dreaded sleep injury (although believe me, it still happens).

Throughout my more than 30 years as a personal fitness trainer, I've trained dozens of clients in their 50s, 60s, 70s, 80s, and even 90s. Not one of them didn't get stronger and improve the quality of their life, even the one who didn't start weight training until she was 87! It is *never too late* to get stronger.

But I will say this: Starting younger *is* better. Yes, you can see benefits from strength training at any age, but your maximum potential to add muscle and get your strongest will decrease the longer you wait to start. You'll never be as young as you are right now. Start *today*, get strong, stay strong!

In the chapters that follow, I'll prove to you not only how beneficial strength training is as we get older, but that it doesn't have to be as complex or as time consuming, or frankly, as *scary*, as some folks make it look.

We'll investigate what's going on with our bodies after 50 and how strength training helps turn back the clock. We'll discuss the foundations of good nutrition and simple, effective strategies to fuel your body like the ageless athlete you are.

Included too are the essential principles to make any weight-training program safe and effective, along with my own favorite exercises and routines that have gotten countless clients of all ages in shape over the last 30 years.

Your goal may not be to look good on camera like Billy, or to withstand the rigors of touring like Stephen or Duff, but you may desire to be strong enough to take a trip to Machu Picchu or feel athletic enough to coach your kid's or grandkid's Little League team.

You might even have competitive aspirations of your own, like my client Barbara Radwin-Garmon (RIP), who started powerlifting in her late 60s after overcoming breast cancer and ultimately won the 2013 IPF World Bench Press Championship at age 70. It's *never* too late!

Personally, and professionally, I have experienced firsthand the rewards of strength training and the empowerment that comes from being strong. The book that follows is my life's work. I share it with you hoping you too will discover the fountain of youth that strength training provides. And always remember that strength never gets old!

CHAPTER 1

The 50-Plus Body

Born between 1965 and 1980, Generation X, aka Gen X, became known as the latchkey generation because we basically had to raise ourselves. In our youth, divorce became more prevalent and single-parent households were commonplace, while dual-parent households found more moms working outside the home than ever before. Thus, no matter the makeup of our families, we Gen Xers were usually left to entertain ourselves after school with little or no adult supervision.

As adults, we seem forever caught in a weird limbo between the Baby Boomers who came before us, who've never paid us much attention, and the generations who came after us, who largely ignore us in spite of their deep desire to co-opt our nostalgic '80s memories as their own. This limbo we inhabit extends to the fitness world as well. While you can find plenty of information on geriatric training for seniors, and infinite 20-something fitness "influencers" targeting younger people on social media, few people are talking to us. We're not kids anymore, but we're not quite seniors yet either. So as a card-carrying member of Gen X, I decided to do something about it and wrote a fitness book just for us.

I sometimes think that this generational invisibility we feel makes us forget just how tough we Gen Xers are! We grew up on a diet of Pop Tarts, Spaghet-tiOs, and hose water. We rode around in cars without seatbelts and in the back of open pickup trucks. We ran around with our friends all day on our bicycles until after dark, but NEVER wore bicycle helmets. OK, maybe these weren't the smartest things, but the benefit of all this unsupervised free time (aka neglect?) was that it instilled in us a self-reliant, independent, "I don't need help" attitude. But despite the moxie our upbringing gave us, we still swore that if we had kids one day, we were going to be more present in their lives (and they were going to wear bicycle helmets!).

Nowadays, we value work-life balance more than prior generations. "We'll show those Boomers!" Unfortunately, the joke was on us, because what we've found is that work-life balance doesn't mean *less work*…it just means we are busier than ever at home too. Gen Xers are stretched VERY thin. Our careers are peaking, with more responsibilities than ever, while at home, many of us who delayed parenthood still have school-aged children. Then there are those of us who started families earlier who now find their adult children living back at home. Others still are raising grandchildren while many of our generation are now caring for aging parents too. Is this what Ferris meant when he said, "Life moves pretty fast"?

Generation X is under *a lot* of stress, and that stress is compounded by the fact that our bodies seem to be betraying us right when we need the most strength and energy possible. We aren't rebounding from injury and illness like we used to, we have aches and pains in places we never even knew we had, and who can get a good night's sleep when we wake up so many times to pee?

Unfortunately, most Americans, especially we "mature" ones, neglect the one activity that could most help to keep us strong, fit, healthy, and able to deal better with all life's stresses: *strength training*. One study found that only 8.9 percent of Americans over age 15 engaged in regular weightlifting, while another study found that 13.7 percent of Americans over the age of 50 practiced regular strength training at least two times a week (Bureau of Labor Statistics 2016; Kruger, Carlson, and Buchner 2007). Perhaps you're already in that nearly 14 percent who regularly resistance trains and are looking to this book for a simple, safe, and effective training program. If so, great…I've got you covered. But if you are one of the vast majority of folks who don't currently strength train, I'll do my best to convince you that *now* is the perfect time to start pumping iron!

Over my career I've heard a common refrain from many older prospective clients: "I'm too old to lift weights." My reply is always the same: "You're too old *not* to lift weights!" We 50-somethings share little in common with our ancestors. As recently as 1920, life expectancy in the United States was barely above 53, so if you made it past 50, you were *old* (Statista 2022). Not anymore! With U.S. life expectancy now averaging 76 years, today's 50-year-olds likely spend little time picking out a casket or wondering if we'll make it to retirement age. And we aren't happy to just be alive—we want to *thrive*!

This combination of living longer and being busier (and more stressed) means we must do everything in our power to stay as strong as we can for as long as we can. Yes, we're busy, but we can't be too busy to take care of our own health and fitness. Want to be able to help your elderly parents and your children and grandchildren? Stay strong. Want to look and feel years if not decades younger (and if the Pitts, Cruises, and Anistons are any indication, we do!)? You guessed it: stay strong.

THE BIG THREE

But what if looking like an ageless celebrity isn't motivating to you. If so, you might consider our need to combat the big three age-related health issues: *sarcopenia*, *metabolism decline*, and *osteoporosis*. While these issues may seem years off and we may still feel like a member of *The Breakfast Club* at heart, we're much closer to retirement than detention. Our 50s are the perfect time to redouble our efforts in the gym, because regular strength training is our best weapon to fight Father Time before it's too late.

Sarcopenia

Sarcopenia is a condition characterized by age-related loss of muscle mass, strength, and function. It affects millions of older adults worldwide and is associated with increased risk of falls, disability, and mortality. Although the exact reasons sarcopenia occurs are not fully understood, it is thought to result from a combination of factors, including changes in hormone levels and function, increased inflammation, and reduced physical activity (Walston 2012). Unfortunately, sarcopenia can begin as early as age 30 and progresses at a rate of 3 to 5 percent per decade, accelerating after age 60 (Volpi, Nazemi, and Fujita 2004). Our 50s are our last best chance to fight sarcopenia, and our weapon is strength training.

Research has shown that strength training is an effective way to combat sarcopenia (Hurst et al. 2022). Strength training promotes muscle growth and preserves muscle mass and function in older adults. A review of 22 randomized controlled trials (RCTs) found that strength training is even more beneficial when combined with protein supplementation, which significantly increased muscle mass, strength, and physical performance in older adults with sarcopenia or frailty (Liao, Tsauo, and Wu 2017).

Another review of 121 RCTs (involving 6,700 participants) found that strength training improved muscle mass, strength, and function in older people with sarcopenia (Liu and Latham 2009). For me, battling sarcopenia simply means staying strong and maintaining my muscle mass as I age, thus keeping my independence and enhancing my personal safety. I strive to be more physically resilient and lessen the impact of accidents or illnesses I may deal with in the future. This in turn helps me to stress less mentally and emotionally about getting older. And yes, I look better in the mirror too!

Metabolism

We've all said it or heard it at some point: "I can't lose weight; I must have a slow metabolism." But is it true, and does it really matter? Metabolism is the energy required to operate and maintain all the processes in the body. We quantify this energy expenditure as calories. In other words, metabolism, or metabolic rate, is how many calories we burn daily.

The bulk of the calories we expend comes from our *basal metabolic rate* (BMR), which is how much energy you burn at rest. This is the part of metabolism that people (perhaps unknowingly) are referring to when they think of slow metabolism. Genetics does play a role in determining whether your metabolic rate is faster or slower, but you can't change your parents. So, focus on what you can change, because the other big factor impacting your BMR is how much muscle mass you have. Even the differences we see in metabolism based on age or sex are largely just differences in muscle mass—for example, males tend to have more muscle mass than females, thus a higher metabolism, and older people tend to have less muscle mass than younger people, hence a slower metabolism.

On top of BMR, three main contributors add to our *total daily energy expenditure* (TDEE). As you may have guessed, exercise is a contributor. But so too is *non-exercise activity thermogenesis* (NEAT). NEAT is how active you are above rest, but not including actual exercise. Think how physical your job is or how many steps you get in daily as a normal part of life.

Last, the *thermic effect of food* (TEF) plays a role. We'll address TEF more in chapter 3, but for now know that TEF means the calories burned to digest, absorb, and use the foods we eat.

Outside of metabolic diseases, age-related slowing of metabolism is a well-documented phenomenon, but it starts much later than we thought previously. A recent study showed that metabolism stays fairly consistent from age 20 to age 60, with an average decrease of 1 percent per year after age 60 (Pontzer et al. 2021). The study analyzed data from over 6,400 people between the ages of eight days and 95 years and found that the metabolic rate peaks in infancy, then steadily declines through childhood and adolescence until adulthood, where it stays relatively constant until age 60.

Overall, the study challenges the common belief that metabolism slows down significantly throughout adulthood and suggests that lifestyle factors such as diet and exercise may have a greater impact on metabolic rate than previously thought. This is great news for us 50-somethings! But if we don't get our proverbial house in order before age 60, age-related slowing of metabolism will exacerbate weight gain and thus increase our risk of type 2 diabetes, heart disease, and stroke.

Strength training and improvements to muscle mass have been shown to mitigate the age-related slowing of metabolism in several ways. First, muscle tissue is more metabolically active than fat tissue, meaning muscle requires more energy to maintain. Thus, adding muscle mass through strength training can help to boost the body's BMR and increase energy expenditure at rest. Studies have shown a 1.4 kilogram (about 3 pounds) increase in muscle mass when older adults trained two to three days a week for 10 to 12 weeks. Each kilogram (2.2 pounds) of added muscle tissue boosts resting metabolism by about 20 calories per day. Perhaps more important, metabolism increases of 7 to 9 percent for up to three days after a training session are seen as the body tries to repair and maintain lean tissue post workout (Westcott 2012; Srikanthan and Karlamangla 2014). Although NEAT is highly variable and can be difficult to measure, it's been found that added muscle is as important for stimulating NEAT as it is for stimulating resting metabolic rate. It's thought the added muscle inherently stimulates spontaneous physical activity (von Loeffelholz and Birkenfeld 2022).

Second, strength training has been shown to improve insulin sensitivity, which is the body's ability to use insulin to transport blood sugar from the bloodstream into the cells for energy. This is important because insulin resistance (the inability for blood sugar to get into cells) is a major risk factor for type 2 diabetes, which is more common in older adults. Studies have shown that improving insulin sensitivity through strength training can help prevent or manage diabetes and other metabolic disorders (Eves and Plotnikoff 2006; Iglay et al. 2007).

Finally, strength training has been shown to improve cardiovascular health, which is important for maintaining metabolic health and reducing the risk of chronic disease. Studies have shown that strength training can improve blood pressure, cholesterol levels, and overall cardiovascular function in older adults (Cornelissen and Smart 2013; Williams and Stewart 2009).

For these reasons, our 50s are our make-or-break decade to add muscle mass (and strength) before age-related metabolic slowdown starts to chip away in our 60s and beyond. If you aren't strength training, *now* is the time to start!

Osteoporosis

Osteoporosis is a disease characterized by low bone mass and deterioration of bone tissue, leading to increased fragility and risk of fractures. It is more common in older adults, particularly women, and is associated with a range of health complications and reduced quality of life.

Strength training has been shown to be an effective way to prevent and manage osteoporosis in several ways. First, strength training involves loading the bones with weight-bearing exercises such as squats, deadlifts, and lunges. This helps to stimulate the bones to become denser and stronger over time. Studies have shown that strength training can lead to significant increases in *bone mineral density* (BMD) in older adults, particularly in the spine and hips, which are common sites of fracture in osteoporosis (Lohman et al. 1995; Martyn-St James and Carroll 2013).

Second, strength training can help improve balance and coordination, which can reduce the risk of falls and fractures in older adults with osteoporosis. Falls are a major driver of fragility fractures, but a consistent strength-and-balance program can improve postural control (Howe et al. 2011) and has been shown to reduce fall incidence by roughly one-third (Sherrington et al. 2019), helping you stay active and independent well into your golden years.

DEALING WITH PAIN AND DISCOMFORT

Luckily, strength training after 50 doesn't have to be much different than in our younger years. The mechanisms that cause our bodies to get stronger and add lean mass are the same. There are no special exercises that an older trainee *must* do or must *never* do—unless a condition or injury excludes a certain exercise—despite fearmongering articles on the internet.

However, that doesn't mean that our bodies haven't changed over the years and that we should train like a college football player. In my younger years I never thought I'd have to adapt how I trained when I got older. I figured if I kept training and stayed strong (which I have), why would I need to make concessions for age? And this was largely true well into my 40s. What I failed to consider was the normal wear and tear my body would experience from both everyday life *and* a lifetime of training. We gym rats often forget that training is a stress on the body. While this is typically a good thing (and how we get our bodies to change), too much stress in the short term can lead to overtraining, and too much training in the long run can increase the risk of overuse injuries.

Unfortunately for me, the cartilage in my knees has slowly worn away, and when I squat heavy and to competition depth (hips below parallel with the knee), I suffer from Baker's cysts. Unsurprisingly, I don't squat heavy to depth anymore. I work around it. In the exercise chapters I'll discuss my favorite alternative exercises for a variety of issues you could be dealing with.

By this age almost all of us are experiencing pain or discomfort somewhere. It could be an old high school sports injury that hurts when you barbell bench press; or that pain in your neck that flares up every time the weather turns cold; or just simple wear and tear from a life well lived. In addition to any preexisting injuries and the big three, we "mature" trainees may also be dealing with other medical issues such as diabetes, high blood pressure, or arthritis, or we are taking medications that can impact our training.

None of these issues are reasons to avoid training, because the benefits of resistance training are far too great to miss out on. But as important as strength training is, you need to be able to incorporate it into your busy schedule efficiently, safely, and consistently to truly benefit from this fountain of youth.

Remember in the introduction when I mentioned the "dreaded sleep injuries"? I was only half joking. The fact is that most of us over 50 do wake up with some kind of ache, pain, or discomfort. That doesn't mean we are "injured" and shouldn't train. At this age, if we only trained on the days when we felt 100 percent, we'd rarely, if ever, train.

My clients hear me say that "some days are diamonds, and some days are coal." Showing up on those "coal days," when you "slept wrong" and just don't feel like training can often be when most of your progress is made. "Diamond days" are simply too rare to count on, so you need to get the most you can out of those coal days.

Of course, if you are truly ill, stay home and rest. And if you are injured, depending on the extent and severity of the injury, you'll likely be able to train around the issue. But if you just feel out of sorts, and dare I say, lazy, go to the gym and see how the warm-up goes. If you feel good after that, try a warm-up set on your first exercise.

If anything causes a sharp pain, stop! But the "general malaise" of small aches and stiffness most of us deal with on the regular will typically go away as we warm up. Remember, although we are always striving to do more reps or lift more weights than our prior workouts, we also don't want to turn a small problem into a big one. If you are unsure how you're feeling after a warm-up set or two, go lighter on your work sets—as light as you need to so you don't exacerbate what you are feeling.

Although we all want to train like a montage from a *Rocky* movie, remember that no rep or set, exercise, or workout is worth an injury that leads to prolonged absence from the gym. Listen to your body and let pain be your guide. Go lighter, skip an exercise altogether, or skip the weights entirely, do some cardio, and live to fight another day.

INFLUENCE OF MEDICATIONS

Several medications that many trainees over 50 are taking can have an impact on strength training. In this section, we will look at some of the most common ones (Healthline 2023; Friedrich 2023; Saleh 2020; Sohal 2023).

Corticosteroids (e.g., Prednisone, Dexamethasone)

These medications, commonly used to treat inflammation, autoimmune disorders, and asthma, can cause muscle wasting (atrophy) and weaken connective tissues. Their use can impact strength training by reducing muscle protein synthesis, increasing catabolism (muscle breakdown), and creating a higher risk of tendon injuries.

Statins (e.g., Atorvastatin, Simvastatin)

Used to lower cholesterol, these medications may cause muscle pain, weakness, and rhabdomyolysis (a severe muscle breakdown condition). Their use can impact strength training by impairing muscle recovery, leading to fatigue and reducing exercise capacity.

Beta-Blockers (e.g., Metoprolol, Propranolol)

Used to treat high blood pressure, heart conditions, and anxiety, beta-blockers reduce heart rate and blood pressure. Their use can impact strength training by lowering exercise endurance, reducing blood flow to muscles, and causing fatigue and dizziness during workouts.

Selective Serotonin Reuptake Inhibitors (SSRIs) (e.g., Fluoxetine, Sertraline)

Used to treat depression and anxiety, some SSRIs can lead to fatigue, drowsiness, and muscle weakness. Their use may impact strength training by reducing power output, slowing reaction time, and increasing risk of injury due to coordination issues.

Benzodiazepines (e.g., Diazepam, Lorazepam)

Prescribed for anxiety, insomnia, and seizures, benzodiazepines can cause sedation, muscle relaxation, and dizziness. Their use may impact strength training by reducing muscle-contraction strength, slowing reaction time, and impairing coordination.

Diuretics (e.g., Furosemide, Hydrochlorothiazide)

Used to treat high blood pressure and fluid retention, diuretics cause water and electrolyte loss. Their use may impact strength training by possibly leading to muscle cramps, dehydration, weakness, and lower endurance.

Antipsychotics (e.g., Risperidone, Olanzapine)

These drugs can cause weight gain, increase fatigue, and affect levels of dopamine, a neurotransmitter essential for motivation and movement. Their use may impact strength training by lowering energy levels, reducing neuromuscular coordination, and increasing risk of metabolic issues.

Chemotherapy Drugs

Used in cancer treatment, chemotherapy drugs often cause muscle loss, fatigue, and joint pain. Their use may impact strength training by reducing muscle mass, weakening bones, and impairing immune function.

Opioids (e.g., Oxycodone, Morphine)

Used for pain relief, opioids can cause drowsiness, muscle relaxation, and reduced motivation. Their use may impact strength training by slowing muscle recovery, decreasing testosterone levels, and increasing injury risk.

Anabolic-Androgenic Steroids (Long-Term Use)

While anabolic steroids increase muscle mass and strength in the short term, long-term use can lead to muscle and tendon weakness, heart issues, and hormonal imbalances. Their use may impact strength training in that they may cause tendon ruptures, joint pain, and long-term muscle damage.

There are ways to minimize the impact of medications on strength training:

- Talk to a doctor about potential alternatives or dosage adjustments.
- Increase protein intake to help counteract muscle loss.
- Stay hydrated if taking diuretics or medications that cause dehydration.
- Monitor fatigue levels and adjust training intensity accordingly.
- Incorporate recovery strategies such as sleep optimization, stretching, and mobility exercises.

WRAPPING UP

As we can see, resistance training is the top weapon in our arsenal in the fight against sarcopenia, metabolic slowdown, and osteoporosis. And by improving and maintaining our muscle mass, we lessen the chance of metabolic-related health problems such as diabetes, heart disease, and stroke.

Understanding the rewards of pumping iron is one thing, but putting it into practice can be quite another. It's easy to hit the gym regularly in our teens and

20s, but when we get older, commitments to family, work, and other areas of interest compete for free time. But as you now know, strength training should be a nonnegotiable part of a healthy lifestyle, especially as we get older. So, let's continue in chapter 2, where we'll discuss the simplest and most effective ways to ensure we make it to the gym and achieve the results we desire both safely and efficiently.

CHAPTER 2

Pillars of Strength Training

Gen Xers, I've got good news! Not only are you not "too old" for strength training, but you don't even have to train as often or as intensely as hundreds of Gen-Z fitness influencers may have led you to believe. Don't get me wrong—if you want the myriad benefits that strength training offers, you *are* going to have to train regularly, but you don't need to do the super high-intensity, leave-you-in-a-puddle-of-sweat (or worse!), grind-you-down-to-a-nub style workout that's become popular in large part due to social media.

Training after age 50 requires a certain amount of finesse, and pushing too hard too often can be detrimental to your training goals. Hyperintense, repetitive workouts can leave you sore, exhausted, and more prone to injury. The life of a busy 50-something is already tough enough; the last thing you need is for your workout to beat you up more than it helps you.

I know you've seen fitness fads come and go and probably participated in a few along the way: the running boom, Jazzercise, step aerobics, the ThighMaster, circuit training, Tae Bo, the Insanity workout, CrossFit, spinning, the Shake Weight, kettlebells, Curves, Peloton, and on and on. With so many options claiming to be "the answer," it can be impossible to know what to do! I understand your frustration.

Fitness trends remind me of a scene from the 1987 teen comedy *Can't Buy Me Love*. A young Patrick Dempsey (long before he became Dr. McDreamy) played nerdy Ronald Miller. Ronald pays cheerleader Cindy Mancini to be his girlfriend for a month to try to make him popular. The ruse works, and Ronald starts to become popular, culminating in him being challenged to perform the latest dance at a school sock hop.

Unfortunately for Ronald, while he thinks he is learning the latest dance from *American Bandstand*, he is actually watching PBS and learning the African anteater ritual. At the dance, Ronald starts gyrating and gesticulating, at first perplexing his fellow students. But quickly they too join in the fray, and the African anteater ritual becomes all the rage at school.

Over my decades as a personal trainer, many of these "anteater rituals" have taken the fitness scene by storm. Fortunately for me, I based my business on solid training principles and didn't change my methods every time a new fitness trend became popular. I'm convinced this is a big reason why I'm still "dancing" and many of those trendy competitors are long gone.

Unfortunately, proper strength training can be somewhat boring and repetitive, so it's no wonder that when something new and shiny comes along promising to help us achieve six-pack abs, a firm booty, or big biceps in just minutes per week, we naturally fall for it . . . again! But these quick fixes are usually unsustainable or just outright gimmickry.

I prefer to compare training to saving money: slow, steady deposits of effort that provide consistent results over time, the "compounding interest" of fitness, if you will. Unfortunately, we humans seem to be hardwired to pursue the quick fix, a lotto ticket investment in our fitness.

We want results, we want them yesterday, and we want our workouts to be both motivating and entertaining, all for a minimum time commitment. So once more we plow headlong into the latest fad and burn out before we've washed our new workout clothes for the second time. Until the next "big thing" comes around. . . .

My goal is to demystify strength training for you and show you how to make regular training safe, effective, and, dare I say it, enjoyable! For me, the choice is obvious: strength train or get old. I'm reminded of the Bruce Springsteen song "Glory Days" . . . if we don't strength train as we age, we'll turn into that boring person who always talks about how much we used to be able to lift "back in the day." I don't know about you, but I'm not satisfied reminiscing about what I "used to do." While strength training can't do anything about our chronological age, it can literally turn back the clock on our biological age.

To illustrate this point, consider the incredible MRI images showing a cross section of the thighs of a 40-year-old triathlete, a sedentary 74-year-old, and a 70-year-old triathlete (figure 2.1) (Piasecki 2019). It's astounding how similar the 40- and 70-year-old triathletes' MRIs look, but more important, how different they look from the sedentary 74-year-old! The sedentary person's legs remind me of old, dry beef jerky with a big rind of fat around it. How different than the hard-training septuagenarian!

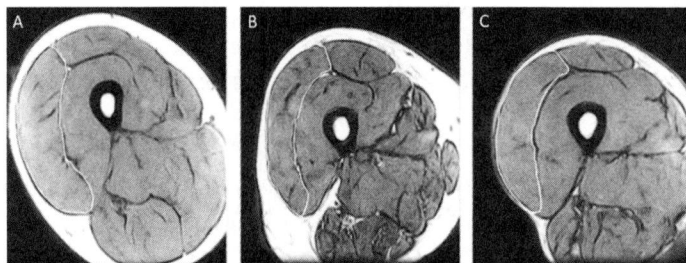

FIGURE 2.1   MRI of thigh muscles.

Reprinted from M. Piasecki, A. Ireland, J. Piasecki, et al. "Long-Term Endurance and Power Training May Facilitate Motor Unit Size Expansion to Compensate for Declining Motor Unit Numbers in Older Age," *Physiologia*, 10 (2019). Distributed under the terms of the Creative Commons Attribution 4.0 International License (http://creaticecommons.org/licenses/by/4.0/).

This one illustration is all the motivation I need to keep training hard for the rest of my life. It reminds me of the big antismoking campaign in schools back in the late '70s. I vividly remember seeing a comparison of the real lungs of a nonsmoker and those of a smoker. The image of the healthy pink lungs of the nonsmoker contrasted with the smoker's hideous black lungs is seared into my memory. There was no chance I would ever smoke after that. The MRI image had the same effect: I'll do everything I can to maintain my muscle mass for the rest of my life!

This doesn't mean we need to become triathletes to fight Father Time. Throughout my decades as a personal trainer, most of my clients have trained with me for two or three days a week and for only one hour each workout. Strength training should be the foundation of your fitness pursuits. The methods I share in this book are the same ones I've used for over 30 years with Hollywood's movers and shakers, and they will be just as effective for you to make strength training consistently doable, regardless of your age or the busyness of your schedule.

CONSISTENCY IS KEY

I have a lot of experience training the 50-plus crowd, and I can say without hesitation that, aside from not training at all, the biggest issue keeping people from achieving their fitness goals is lack of consistency.

While true at any age, I find it imperative that older trainees stay consistent with their workout programs. The phrase "use it or lose it" could not be any truer the older we get. We might be able to get away with training randomly or not much at all when we are younger, but as we saw in chapter 1, sarcopenia and osteoporosis are coming for us, and to fight them we need consistent, progressive strength training.

In my mid-50s, I am able to compete in bench press competitions against athletes half my age. I currently train several clients in their 50s, 60s, and 70s who are strong and robust and who defy their calendar age. But perhaps my greatest examples for the power of strength training for older adults come from my oldest and longest-term clients.

My oldest client was 95 years old. Doris didn't start training until she was 87 when, according to her daughters, she "started to slow down a little." She trained twice a week with me for 8 years and was able to improve her strength even into her 90s. One of my biggest goals for her was to be strong enough to never get stranded on a low public toilet, which happened to my own grandmother. Not only did this never happen to my client, but even during the last days of her life, she was able to get up and take herself to the bathroom. No bedpan necessary. Death with dignity. The power of strength training.

One of my longest-term clients, Barbara, trained with me for 25 years from age 51 to age 76 when she passed away. She not only got stronger with age but was able to recover from severe crippling injuries AND breast cancer to win the World Bench Press Championship at 70 years of age after doctors told her she'd never regain full use of her left hand and that she should never lift more than 5 or 10 pounds ever again. The power of strength training.

To achieve life-empowering results like these, consistency of training is paramount. Let's look at several strategies that encourage it.

Avoid Injury

First and foremost, we need to avoid injury. Nothing is as big a progress and motivation killer as needing to take days, weeks, or even months off from training due to injury. But many of us are so desperate for change that we jump into training too hard and too fast, mistaking intensity as being the most important thing. If we're lucky, we "just" get debilitatingly sore, and if we're not so lucky, we get injured. There goes our consistency!

By age 50, many of us are coping with the remnants of old injuries and need our training programs to help these old aches and pains feel better, not add to our misery. We will likely need to train around and slowly through these issues to make progress. But while training too intensely too soon isn't the way to go, not training our muscles at all for fear of injury, and thus becoming even weaker, isn't a great alternative.

Aside from taking care not to overdo it when training, other critical injury-prevention strategies include choosing exercises with a lower risk of injury and using proper form on the exercises we do use. Resist the temptation to mimic the "parlor tricks" you see on social media. You don't need to do high box jumps or try squatting while balancing on a Swiss ball or anything else where the risk far outweighs the reward. Don't try to be the Evel Knievel of the weight room. Train sensibly, train consistently, and avoid injuries, period.

Be Realistic and Patient

Unrealistic expectations can also cripple consistency. Many of us, especially those who used to be in shape, set ourselves up for failure before we even start. You may have been in great shape in high school or college, but if you haven't been training for some time or have been inconsistent at best, do yourself a favor and forget what you used to do. Start light, progress slowly, and avoid injury while you reclaim your body from Father Time.

That doesn't mean you can't get as strong as you used to be. Heck, you might even surpass your previous bests. I didn't achieve a 300-pound bench press until I was nearly 50. I was close back in my 20s, but I didn't listen to my shoulder when it started to complain. I ended up injuring myself while attempting a 285-pound bench. The difference now is that I listen to my body and am patient. Give yourself time. Don't be in a rush. We are playing the long game here. Remember, if you get hurt, you aren't going to be consistent, and if you aren't consistent, you aren't going to see results. Patience, grasshopper!

TRAINING SMARTER

I know I said lack of consistency is the biggest problem, and for those who haven't been training, it is, but we self-motivated 50-somethings who have stayed active often have the opposite problem—we train too hard, too long, too often. Our intentions are good, but our execution is flawed. While it's completely understandable to want to train as hard and as frequently as in our younger years, we simply aren't that young anymore, and if we don't include some caveats with our training, we'll end up injured and inconsistent, just like a neophyte lifter.

The fitness industry is dominated by younger individuals. The average age of a personal trainer in the United States is 37 (Zippia 2023), and 54 percent of influencers on Instagram are between the ages of 25 and 34, with another 34 percent *under* the age of 25 (Hutchinson 2019). I don't know about you, but even though I've been training hard my entire life, my body reacts differently now that I'm over 50. Even the best young personal trainer has no idea what 50 feels like, and the worst fitness influencers think we're all Boomers and should stay out of the gym so we don't get in the way of their videos.

Gen Z's fitness recommendations often focus on things that are inappropriate for our physical abilities or our place in life. "No, Kyle, I don't have time to lift four days a week and do cardio every day and prep all my meals for the week on Sunday and get eight hours of sleep in a hyperbaric chamber every night and practice my sun salutations in the morning . . ." You get my drift.

Many training programs, though well intentioned, are too convoluted and time consuming, with sessions lasting 90 minutes or more including a general warm-up, dynamic warm-up, prehab, activation, and then, if there's time, the actual workout. That isn't to say those things don't have value, but I've found that older trainees need a program that gets them *strong*, and we rarely have the time to do the "extras" that a 22-year-old influencer, who has all day to train (and post about it online) does. And too often young trainers have the mindset that someone their parents' age needs to be treated with kid gloves, so they focus on a lot of submaximal "busywork" and never have the trainee actually lift heavy things.

Yes, strength training at any age does have inherent risk of injury, but as mature trainees we can minimize these risks in several ways:

1. Don't train too frequently: Two or three lifting days a week is fine for most of us.
2. Don't train for too long in any single session: 40 to 60 minutes should do it.
3. Train heavy but not too heavy (see the Intensity section later in this chapter).
4. Don't perform a risky exercise if a safer one exists.
5. Get adequate sleep: Seven to nine hours is a good goal.
6. Use proper nutrition to enhance recovery after workouts (see chapter 3).

Aside from making our workouts safer, what can we do to maximize our progress in the gym? The following are principles I use in designing strength-training programs that should help you design your own programs after you exhaust the ones in this book.

TRAINING PRINCIPLES

Although my clients like that they can just show up and not think about their workouts because I handle it all, I still like to explain why I have them do things a certain way. Then, if they ever have to train without me, they can do so intelligently and safely. And if you're reading this book, you likely will be training on your own, and I want you to know as much about the what, why, and how of training programs as my clients do.

Strength Training Fundamentals

Progressive overload is the overarching principle of strength training. As the name implies, to progress, we must consistently try to do more than we've done in previous workouts. During my days in public gyms, I saw far too many fitness enthusiasts do the exact same exercises with the exact same weight for the same number of sets and reps, week after week, year after year, and wonder why their physiques never changed. In this instance, consistency is not enough. We need to try to progress by lifting more sets and reps with the same weight or adding more weight. Without progressive overload, you will not change your body or get stronger.

The SAID principle (*specific adaptations to imposed demands*) is a fancy way of saying that your body will adapt based on the demands you place on it. So, since we are trying to build muscle and strength, we need workouts designed to do specifically that. We shouldn't try to use endurance-type workouts (even those that use weights) to get bigger and stronger. We'll do a deep dive on the specifics in chapter 10.

Delayed onset muscle soreness, or DOMS, the pain that usually starts a day or two after a hard workout, is something we've all felt. If you've been consistent in the gym, you may not get DOMS very often anymore, and that's OK. While it's common when starting out or trying a new exercise or a heavier weight for the first time, a lack of muscle soreness does *not* mean you didn't have a good or effective workout. I rarely get sore unless I've been sick and had an extended layoff from the gym. This degree of soreness will likely go away during the next workout, if not before. If you are sore for several days, you likely overdid it. Make a note in your training journal and ease off a bit on the next workout or take an extra rest day as needed.

And speaking of a training journal, if you aren't keeping a record of what you've done in the gym and then referring back to it at future workouts to try and beat those prior numbers, you are just guessing at whether you're achieving your goals. I'll go into the use of a training journal in chapter 10.

Athleticism encompasses strength, endurance, and flexibility. This book is focused on strength, but in my opinion, strength training done correctly will also improve endurance (to a degree) and flexibility (if using a full range of motion on exercises). I don't think that the converse is true of endurance or flexibility training. Strength training is the cake, and endurance and flexibility are the frosting and decorations. Focus on the cake.

Categorizing Exercises

Exercises may be categorized by body part, by compound or isolation, and by plane of motion.

The most obvious way to categorize exercises is by body part. We tend to label exercises as chest, back, arms, legs, calves, abs, and so on, and these can be further divided. Chest becomes upper or lower chest; back can be lats, midback, or traps; and legs can be quads or hamstrings.

Compound exercises involve multiple joints and multiple muscle groups; isolation exercises focus on one muscle spanning one joint (with a few exceptions). Using an incline bench press as an example, you could label it a chest exercise or an upper chest exercise. But there are other muscles involved too—triceps and anterior deltoids are worked very hard on this "chest" exercise. If you were trying to isolate the upper chest, you'd choose something like an incline dumbbell fly to minimize assistance from the triceps.

Kinesiology divides the body into three planes: *sagittal, frontal,* and *transverse.* Sagittal divides us into left and right halves, frontal into front and back halves, and transverse into top and bottom halves. Most exercises are sagittal plane exercises because they are forward and backward movements in that sagittal plane;

think flexion and extension. Frontal plane exercises are rarer because they involve side-to-side motions like a lateral lunge or side shuffle. Transverse plane exercises are rotational and involve the spine, shoulders, or hips. An exercise like the bench press can have both sagittal and transverse plane motion. Then there is the scapular plane, which sits about 30 to 40 degrees in front of the frontal plane. It is often beneficial to do shoulder exercises like overhead pressing and lateral raises in this scapular plane because the risk of joint pain or impingement is lessened.

I and many other coaches like to categorize exercises by a simpler system. We think of exercises as vertical push and pull, horizontal push and pull, hip-dominant leg exercises, and quad-dominant leg exercises. Then we may sprinkle in exercises for the biceps, triceps, calves, and abs. And depending on the angle of push or pull, there are exercises I consider hybrid because they are neither truly horizontal or vertical. You can treat them as their own thing or cycle them in on a vertical or horizontal day.

Frequency

Most training programs use *frequency* to mean how many days per week you train, and in this book, we mean weight training. The bulk of my programs are two or three days per week of full-body workouts. This ensures that each body part gets trained multiple times weekly instead of just once, as is the case on many body-part split programs.

Duration and Volume

Duration simply means the length of each training session. Although most of my training sessions take 40 to 60 minutes to complete, there are times when you'll run longer than 60 minutes. Conversely, if you don't have time to train at least 40 minutes, a shorter workout is still beneficial. I'd much rather you do a 10- or 15-minute workout than skip it altogether. If all your workouts tend to be brief, you'll probably be able to train more frequently because each one will be easier to recover from.

Volume means the total reps completed during a workout. If the weights are light and the rest periods are brief, it's possible to accumulate a good amount of volume even if the workout is short. Volume is also entwined with intensity. Some people include the weights used (intensity) as a component of volume. I like to think of them separately and then multiply them to get "total work."

Intensity

Intensity means how much weight was lifted and is often expressed as a percentage of the *one-repetition max* or 1RM (the heaviest weight you can lift one time using good form on a given exercise). For most recreational gym-goers, I do not recommend testing your 1RM. Unless you compete in powerlifting or Olympic weightlifting, there is no need to try a 1RM. In my opinion, the risk of injury is too high, and I don't need to know those numbers to ensure that someone is getting stronger. All I care about is progression. Are you lifting more weight than last workout? Lifting the same weight but for more reps? The same weight and reps but with better form? All these show progress. I simply try to beat last workout's numbers or at least match them with even better form. Yes, it's really that simple.

This is true whether I'm utilizing heavier weights for lower reps or lighter weights for higher reps. Just keep in mind the intensity–volume relationship: the heavier you lift, the fewer reps you'll be able to perform. Conversely, if you prefer higher rep ranges (more volume), you'll need to use lighter weights. This doesn't need to be overthought; just follow the rep recommendations in the next several paragraphs.

Common wisdom regarding reps, or more specifically, rep ranges, used to be that low reps (1 to 5) were for strength only, medium range reps (6 to 12) were for hypertrophy (muscle growth), and high reps (15 to 20) were for fat loss. It's now believed that as long as we are working close to failure—that is, we have no reps left in us—it doesn't matter much what rep range we use. This makes programming workouts much simpler (and dare I say safer) for those of us who are over 50.

The caveat is that we need to be training close to failure regardless of the intensity (weight) or volume (reps) used. Except for the bench press (because I am still a competitive powerlifter), I usually prefer to do at least 8 reps, but more commonly 10 to 15 reps on most exercises. As I've gotten older (and stronger), my joints don't like the constant stress of the heavier weights I'd use in lower rep ranges. To ensure that I'm training with enough intensity (heavy enough), I determine my *reps in reserve* (RIR), which is another way of thinking about my *rate of perceived exertion* (RPE).

Table 2.1 outlines a way to determine reps in reserve.

TABLE 2.1 Reps in Reserve

Rating	Perception	Reps in reserve
0	Maximum effort	0
0.5	Maybe could have done 1 more rep	1
1	Definitely could have done 1 more rep	1
1.5	Definitely could have done 1 more rep; maybe could have done 2 more reps	1-2
2	Definitely could have done 2 more reps	2
2.5	Definitely could have done 2 more reps; maybe could have done 3 more reps	2-3
3	Definitely could have done 3 more reps	3
3.5	Definitely could have done 3 more reps; maybe could have done 4 more reps	3-4
4	Definitely could have done 4 more reps	4
4.5	Definitely could have done 4 more reps; maybe could have done 5 more reps	4-5
5+	Definitely could have done 5 more reps or even more	5+

While training to failure (0 reps in reserve) is not necessary, and could leave you more open to injury, many trainees (both rookie and experienced) don't train heavy enough.

My friend Greg Nuckols wrote an excellent piece (Nuckols 2023) detailing multiple studies showing that the average lifter gravitated toward using about

50 percent of their 1RM for 10 reps. Even those who tested their 1RM prior to the study still chose to lift weights at about 55 percent of their true 1RM.

This is way too low intensity (too light) to stimulate much in the way of strength or hypertrophy improvement. Greg speculates that loads like these may leave up to 10 reps in reserve—10! So in this instance, the trainee needs to either increase the load so they have 1 or 2 RIR left when they hit 10 reps, *or* they need to take that same load to a true 1 or 2 RIR, likely 18 or 19 reps. Again, this shows the relationship between volume and intensity. If the intensity is less (lighter weight), you will need to do more volume (reps) to achieve the desired RIR.

I prefer most sets to be performed with 1 or 2 reps in reserve but will have clients push themselves to a 0.5 or even 0 RIR on final sets of an exercise, particularly if it seems like their RIR on earlier sets might have been a bit more than 1 or 2. But I still want these "hard" reps to have good form.

Exercise Selection

While I do my best to avoid classifying exercises as bad, good, safe, or unsafe, there are exercises that may not be an ideal choice for everyone or at least in certain situations (e.g., when recovering from an injury). Take the barbell bench press, for example. While I love the exercise, I don't think it's the ideal choice for most older clients, especially those with preexisting shoulder injuries. Machines, dumbbells, and cables all provide a similar stimulus to the muscles of the chest, shoulders, and triceps.

My recommendation is to get stronger with machines and bodyweight exercises first and then experiment with the barbell exercises if you're so inclined. But always let pain be your guide. Never perform an exercise that causes sharp pain in the muscles or joints. Sharp pains are not the same as the burn you feel when lifting normally. The exercises in this book will give you many options and progressions that will help you meet your goals while minimizing the potential for injury.

Rest

Polls show that the average American sleeps less than seven hours a night, yet most experts recommend seven to nine hours nightly. In addition, older adults often suffer from poor sleep quality. Our sleeping patterns change, we may not sleep as deeply, and it can take us longer to fall asleep. Not to mention that we often wake up one or more times during the night.

A lack of sleep won't just make us feel sluggish, it's also linked to health issues such as weight gain, diabetes, heart disease, and stroke. People who exercise regularly may need more sleep to recover from workouts than their peers who don't exercise. Fortunately, studies have shown that those who weight train actually improve their sleep duration (Kovacevic et al. 2018). Rest is also important *during* workouts, which we'll discuss in depth in chapter 10.

Nutrition

It shouldn't come as a surprise that good nutrition goes hand in hand with exercise. Food is the fuel that gives us the energy and raw materials for all the processes of the body. And too much or too little fuel can lead to a host of health problems. Proper nutrition is crucial to fuel our workouts and help our bodies recover afterward.

Entire textbooks are devoted to nutrition, but for the purposes of this book, we want simple, actionable advice you can easily implement to help you train hard, recover from workouts, and lead the leaner, healthier, stronger life you desire. So let's head to chapter 3 and uncover the foundations of proper nutrition.

CHAPTER 3

Your Unique Nutritional Needs

Welcome to the nutrition chapter of *Building Strength and Muscle After 50*! When it comes to keeping your body performing optimally as you age like a fine wine, nutrition plays a crucial role. We've come a long way since the 1980s, when fitness and nutrition advice often seemed like it was plucked straight from a sci-fi flick. Let's dive into what you need to know to fuel your strength-training journey in your golden years with science-based evidence recommendations from Angela Dufour, registered sports dietitian.

What's the deal with nutrition once you hit the big 5-0? Well, one thing's for sure: Your body isn't the same as it was back when neon leg warmers were all the rage. You might find that your calorie needs have taken a bit of a nosedive thanks to a lower resting energy expenditure. But fear not—we're not about to let that slow you down.

CALORIE AND MACRONUTRIENT NEEDS

Now, I'm not going to throw a bunch of numbers at you because, hey, we don't eat numbers, we eat delicious food! But it is worth noting that as we age, our bodies tend to need a bit less energy overall. It's all about finding that sweet spot where you're fueling your workouts while meeting your exact nutrition and energy needs and not under- or overdoing it.

When it comes to macronutrients (or macros, as they are commonly called)—carbs, protein, and fat—there's no one-size-fits-all answer to how much of each you need. It really depends on the exact type, time, and intensity of your exercise and what makes you feel your best to meet your overall fitness goals. Just remember, carbs are your body's preferred fuel source, protein helps repair and build muscle, and fat keeps things running smoothly. And don't forget about ample fluids as well. (No, alcohol does not count, but tea and coffee do to a certain extent, but we will get to that.)

Let's break down total energy, macronutrients, and fluid requirements in a bit more detail. Many over 50 complain of weight gain despite following the same

Angela Dufour

Angela C. Dufour has been working as a high-performance certified lead sports dietitian in the Canadian sport system, including the Canadian Sports Institute Atlantic, the Canadian Olympic and Paralympic Sport Institute Network, the Canadian Olympic Committee, and the Professional Women's Hockey League Canada for the past 20 years. She leads a national directive on sport supplement policy, provisions, tracking, and education in Canada with Own the Podium and is a part-time facility instructor at Mount Saint Vincent University in Halifax, Nova Scotia, in the department of applied human nutrition.

Angela graduated with her masters in adult education and a diploma in sports nutrition from the International Olympic Committee in 2007 and is a level 2 anthropometrist, certified by the International Society for the Advancement of Kinathropometry. She is currently pursuing her PhD at the School of Health at the University of the Sunshine Coast, Australia. Angela's research is in the area of food service provisions to improve athletes' health and safety at international sporting competitions. She is the proud mom of a busy 13-year-old boy and can often be found in the rink for work or fueling her son's hockey team.

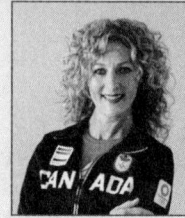

nutritional patterns they did in previous years. Weight gain may be attributed to changes in *resting metabolic rate* (RMR), which entails 60 to 75 percent of an individual's total daily energy expenditure. RMR decreases by about 10 percent from early childhood to adulthood and another 10 percent from adulthood to the age of retirement. Although there may be changes to what you used to do in terms of types and intensities of sport, several factors have been shown to directly influence RMR, including thyroid hormones, genetics, body or environmental temperature, and stress. Other factors related to RMR are body surface area, total body weight, lean body mass, gender, age, and aerobic fitness. Of these factors, there seems to be the strongest correlation between lean body mass and RMR (Tzankoff and Norris 1977). When metabolically active muscle tissue is lost and replaced with metabolically inert depot fat, RMR inevitably declines. By no fault of our own, as we lose lean muscle mass, our RMR will naturally decline, and we will require less total energy compared to our earlier years.

But lucky for you, science has advanced so much in the area of macronutrient needs of the aging active population, that we now know we can fight muscle loss (sarcopenia) and work to keep that RMR as revved up as possible. How do we do that? By making sure that our total energy intake is balanced with our needs. This means adequate intake of carbohydrates, protein, and fats and preventing what the science-y folks call *relative energy deficiency in sport* (REDs). This happens when a mismatch between dietary energy intake and energy expended in exercise leaves the body's total energy needs unmet; that is, there is inadequate energy to support the functions required by the body to maintain optimal health and performance, otherwise known as *low energy availability* (LEA). In other words, energy availability is the dietary energy left over and available for optimal function of body systems (including fueling the RMR!) after accounting for the energy expended from exercise.

Many of you must be thinking, *Well, I was always told that less in, more out will help me lose weight* (if that is your goal). And that is true to a certain extent, until that demand for energy becomes greater than the energy in and leaves little left to support those regular processes. In fact, when athletes are in LEA, the body has a unique way of preserving body fat to protect itself, and folks can end up with a body composition other than what they intended when they lowered their total calorie intake. So, be sure to connect with a registered sports dietitian to determine your *exact* calorie needs to support your strength training if losing weight and body fat is something you desire. Fortunately, RMR can be kept elevated in over-50 individuals who continue to train at high levels while meeting individual nutritional needs. In most individuals, RMR seems to be positively affected by endurance training coupled with resistance training to boost RMR.

Need for Carbohydrates

Now let's talk about where the majority of those calories should be coming from. I know we are in an era of "carbophobes," but if you are active and involved in regular strength training, your body requires energy to come from carbohydrates. *Yes*, all kinds of carbohydrates: simple, complex, fiber (maybe more as we age!). While it is true that our glycogen (the usable form of carbs for energy) storage decreases per unit of muscle as we age, following exercise, older athletes are able to increase muscle glycogen stores and restore glucose postexercise at rates similar to younger athletes. So what does that mean? It means we need to make sure that the timing and amount of our carbs is accurate! Good-quality carbohydrate foods that are supportive of weight management and digestive health and are beneficial for those experiencing chronic disease include oats, grainy breads, brown rice, legumes, and starchy vegetables.

Carbohydrate intake must be periodized according to the type, intensity, and volume of the work you're doing. Refer to table 3.1 to see where you would fit based on your current exercise situation. This can range from low daily amounts (less than 2.5 grams per kilogram of body weight per day or approximately 1.13 grams per pound of body weight per day) on resting or easy training days up to high and very high amounts (greater than 8-10 grams per kilogram of body weight per day or 3.63 to 4.54 grams per pound of body weight per day) on high-intensity training or competition days. Attention should be given to high carbohydrate availability before, during, and after high-intensity training sessions to allow high energy supply and high exercise intensity.

TABLE 3.1   Carb Needs

Daily training schedule	1 hour or less daily activity	1-2 hours daily activity	2-4 hours pretraining	During strength training if training for 1 hour or more	Within 1 hour post strength training
Carbohydrate (55%-70% of total calorie intake)	2-3 g/lb (4.4-6.6 g/kg) body weight per day	3-4 g/lb (6.6-8.8 g/kg) body weight per day	1-1.5g/lb (2.2-3.3 g/kg) body weight	30-40 g/hour	1-1.5g/lb (2.2-3.3 g/kg) body weight

Retain Muscle With Protein

Feel like you are losing muscle in your golden years? You're not imagining it! It has been well reported that as we age, we have a gradual decline in skeletal muscle mass of around 6 to 8 percent per decade after the age of 30 (Janssen et al. 2000; Louis et al. 2019). Fortunately, we *can* use nutrition to combat this, especially if you're strength training to help minimize the loss and promote gains.

It has been suggested that as we age and continue to be active, our needs will be at least 1.2 grams to 2 grams of protein per kilogram of body weight per day with a focus on 35 to 40 grams of leucine-rich protein foods (beef, tofu, milk, soy beverage, whey powder) after strenuous exercise. So for an average 70 kilogram (154-pound) athlete, that's 84 to 149 grams of protein per day. But it isn't enough to get that in a 20-ounce steak! Attention to timing, distribution, and the quality of protein intake is important. That means you should aim for good-quality protein sources (mainly containing leucine amino acid) evenly distributed throughout the day (every 3-4 hours) and in good proportion (minimum 30 grams or at least 0.4 grams per kilogram of body weight [or 0.2 g per pound of body weight] per meal or snack) to maximally stimulate muscle protein synthesis. This corresponds to a minimum of four portions of 30 grams or more of protein per day, for breakfast (at 8 a.m.), lunch (12 p.m.), afternoon snack (4 p.m.), and dinner (8 p.m.) for a total of around 120 grams of protein, or 1.7 grams per kilogram of body mass per day for an 70 kilogram (154-pound) athlete. Care should be taken with protein intakes for people with impaired kidney function, which sometimes occurs in type 2 diabetes.

As you consider what foods to eat to meet your protein needs, remember that not all proteins are created equal. As we age, it becomes more important to prioritize high-quality protein sources that provide all the essential amino acids necessary for muscle repair and growth. Let's dive into the specifics.

Quality of Proteins and Amino Acids

First, let's talk about amino acids. These are the building blocks of protein; I like to call them the Lego of muscle building. There are a total of 20 amino acids (different sizes and colors of Lego blocks) that when combined make whole proteins. Eleven of these different Lego blocks (amino acids) are nonessential, meaning that the body makes them. There are nine essential amino acids that the body cannot produce on its own and must be obtained through diet. These essential amino acids are crucial for muscle protein synthesis, repair, and maintenance, especially during and after strength training. Animal proteins such as meat, poultry, fish, eggs, and dairy from cows are considered complete proteins because they contain all nine essential amino acids in the right proportions. This makes them highly effective for supporting muscle growth and recovery.

While most plant-based protein sources are considered incomplete, meaning they lack one or more essential amino acids, there are a few exceptions. Here are some examples of plant-based complete protein sources:

- **Quinoa:** Quinoa is a versatile pseudograin that is not only rich in protein but also contains all nine essential amino acids. It's an excellent choice for individuals following a vegetarian or vegan diet.
- **Soy:** Soybeans and soy products such as tofu, tempeh, and edamame are complete protein sources. These foods are not only high in protein but also are packed with other nutrients like fiber, vitamins, and minerals.

You can also combine different plant protein sources such as beans, legumes, nuts, seeds, and grains to create complete protein meals that provide all essential amino acids.

Timing of Proteins and Amino Acids

Now, let's talk more about timing. Consuming protein-rich foods or supplements around the time of strength-training sessions can optimize muscle protein synthesis and enhance muscle recovery.

- **Preworkout:** Three to four hours prior to your strength-training session, consuming a protein-rich snack or meal with carbohydrates can provide the body with the necessary amino acids and energy to fuel workouts effectively. This could be a homemade smoothie with fruit and milk or yogurt, Greek yogurt with granola, or a turkey sandwich on whole-grain bread. But the focus should not be taken away from the importance of carbohydrates in the preworkout snack, especially if you only have one hour or less to get a snack in. In this case little protein is needed, and the major macro should be easily digested carbohydrates such as fruit or pretzels.

- **Postworkout:** To counteract the reduced muscle recovery capacity observed in masters athletes, a protein-rich snack is recommended in the immediate postexercise recovery period (i.e., within the first hour). The best protein sources to promote muscle protein synthesis are those containing essential amino acids, leucine in particular. Leucine is well known for its role as a precursor of muscle protein synthesis, and quantities are highest in dairy products and whey protein powders. Many studies have reported the greater effects of whey protein, which is rapidly absorbed and digested, compared to slower proteins such as casein and soy proteins on postexercise muscle protein synthesis rates (Louis et al. 2019; Tang et al. 2009).

Aim for a combination of protein and carbohydrates in the ratio of 1:3 protein to carbs, with a minimum of 25 to 35 grams of quality protein (table 3.2). That's a snack with approximately 30 grams of protein and 90 grams of carbs to replenish glycogen stores and support optimal muscle repair. This could be a homemade protein shake with Greek yogurt, milk, fruit, oats, and hemp hearts, a chicken and quinoa salad, or a tofu stir-fry with rice and vegetables.

TABLE 3.2 Protein Needs

Daily training schedule	1 hour or less daily activity	1-2 hours daily activity	2-4 hours pre-training	During strength training if training for 1 hour or more	Within 1 hour post strength training
Protein (12%-15% of total calorie intake)	0.55 g/lb (1.2 g/kg) body weight per day	0.65 g/lb (1.4 g/kg) body weight per day	0.15-0.25 g/lb (0.3-0.6 g/kg) body weight	None needed	0.25-0.35 g/lb (0.6-0.8 g/kg) body weight

Can You Get Too Much Protein?

It is possible to consume too much protein, regardless of age. While protein is essential for muscle repair, immune function, and various other physiological processes, excessive protein intake can have potential risks and adverse effects, especially as we age. Here are some of the risks associated with excess protein consumption:

- **Kidney strain:** Excessive protein intake can put strain on the kidneys, as they are responsible for filtering and excreting waste products, such as urea and ammonia, from protein metabolism. Over time, this increased workload may contribute to decreased kidney function and exacerbate preexisting kidney conditions.

- **Dehydration:** High-protein diets can increase the body's need for water to help flush out the byproducts of protein metabolism. Inadequate hydration can lead to dehydration, which can strain the kidneys and impair overall health and well-being, particularly in older adults who may already be at increased risk of dehydration due to age-related changes in thirst perception and kidney function.

- **Digestive issues:** Consuming large amounts of protein, especially from certain sources such as whey or casein supplements, may lead to digestive discomfort such as bloating, gas, and diarrhea. Older adults may be more susceptible to digestive issues due to age-related changes in digestion and absorption.

- **Bone health:** Some research suggests that high-protein diets may be associated with increased calcium excretion and reduced calcium absorption, which could potentially have negative implications for bone health, particularly in individuals at risk of osteoporosis (Kerstetter, O'Brien, and Insogna 2003). However, more studies are needed to fully understand the impact of protein intake on bone health, especially in older adults.

- **Nutrient imbalances:** Focusing too heavily on protein-rich foods or supplements may lead to imbalances in other essential nutrients, such as carbohydrates, fats, vitamins, and minerals. A well-rounded diet that includes a variety of nutrient-dense foods is essential for overall health and well-being, especially as we age and our nutritional needs may change.

The bottom line for you over-50 muscle buffs is to prioritize high-quality protein sources that provide all essential amino acids to support muscle health and recovery. Whether from animals or plants, protein-rich foods consumed before and after workouts can optimize muscle protein synthesis and promote overall well-being. Remember to consult with a registered dietitian for personalized nutrition recommendations based on individual health needs and fitness goals.

Choose the Right Fats

Fat recommendations for golden gymmers are similar to those for the general population, with some considerations for age-related changes in metabolism and overall health. Lower carbohydrate, higher fat diets have become the rage in popular fitness social media, and while they have been shown to promote adaptations such as enhanced fat oxidation during exercise, they generally lead to impaired ability to utilize carbohydrate for high-intensity efforts (Burke et al. 2017).

Here are some key points to keep in mind:

- **Prioritize healthy fats.** Focus on consuming monounsaturated and polyunsaturated fats, which have been shown to have numerous health benefits, including supporting heart health, reducing inflammation, and improving cognitive function. This is particularly important for our older athletes with cardiovascular disease or those at higher risk of cardiovascular disease (e.g., people with type 2 diabetes). Sources of healthy fats include avocados, nuts and seeds (e.g., almonds, walnuts, chia seeds), plant-based oils, fatty fish (e.g., salmon, mackerel, trout), flaxseeds and flaxseed oil, and nut butters (e.g., peanut butter, almond butter).

- **Limit saturated and trans fats.** While some saturated fats are OK in moderation, it's essential to limit intake of saturated and trans fats because they have been linked to increased risk of heart disease and other chronic health conditions. Sources of saturated and trans fats include red meat, full-fat dairy products, processed meats (e.g., bacon, sausage), fried foods, and margarine and other partially hydrogenated oils.

- **Consider omega-3 fatty acids.** Omega-3 fatty acids are essential for heart health, brain function, and reducing inflammation. They are found primarily in fatty fish (use the acronym SMAASHTT to remember the fattiest of fatty fish: salmon, mackerel, arctic char, anchovies, sardines, herring, trout, tuna), but are also found in walnuts, flaxseeds, and chia seeds. Including sources of omega-3 fats in your diet can help support overall health and may also aid in recovery and muscle repair after strength-training workouts. (See supplements section for more details.)

- **Monitor total fat intake.** While fats are an essential part of a healthy diet, they are also calorie dense, so it's important to monitor your overall fat intake, especially if you're trying to manage your weight. Pay attention to portion size and aim to incorporate fats into your meals and snacks in moderation. But don't be fat-phobic! Consuming less than your recommended amount (less than 20 percent of your total energy intake) may compromise fat-soluble vitamins (A, D, E, K). A general rule of thumb is aim for 0.5 grams per pound (1-1.5 grams per kilogram) of body weight per day.

Get Enough Fluids

Fluids are crucial for maintaining hydration, supporting performance, and promoting overall health and well-being. Individual fluid needs can vary based on body size, sweat rate, climate, and exercise intensity. Age-related changes such as decreased perception of thirst, decreased kidney function, changes in hormones, and changes in sweat response may mean decreased voluntary fluid intake during exercise or increased requirements. Also, if you're exercising in hot or humid conditions or for prolonged periods, you may need to increase your fluid intake to compensate for greater sweat losses. Here are some general fluid recommendations:

- First, stay hydrated. Aim to drink water regularly throughout the day, not just during workouts. Thirst is not always a reliable indicator of hydration, especially in older adults, so it's important to drink fluids consistently to prevent dehydration. Pay attention to your urine color; pale yellow urine is a sign of adequate hydration, while dark yellow urine may indicate dehydration.

- For your pre-workout hydration, drink 16 to 20 ounces (about 500 to 600 milliliters) of water two to three hours before exercise to ensure adequate hydration status. Consume an additional 8 to 10 ounces (about 250 to 300 milliliters) of water 10 to 20 minutes before starting your workout.

• During strength-training sessions, aim to drink water regularly to replace fluids lost through sweat. Sip on water between sets or during rest periods. If workouts last longer than 60 minutes or occur in hot and humid conditions, consider consuming a sports drink that contains electrolytes to replace lost fluids and electrolytes.

• After exercise, drink fluids to replace losses incurred during the workout. Aim to consume 16 to 24 ounces (about 500 to 700 milliliters) of water for every pound (0.5 kilograms) of body weight lost during exercise.

• Watch out for signs of dehydration, such as dry mouth, dark urine, fatigue, dizziness, and headache. If you experience any of these symptoms, increase your fluid intake immediately.

• Have a hydration plan! Measurements of fluid needs through pre- and posttraining and competition weights are recommended to help determine fluid requirements for individual athletes.

MICRONUTRIENT NEEDS

Now, on to the little guys, the vitamins and minerals that keep your body functioning like a well-oiled machine. As we age, some of these nutrients might need a bit more attention. For example, vitamin D becomes extra important for maintaining bone health since our bones tend to get a bit cranky as we get older.

Much remains to be learned about the effects of aging and activity on vitamin and mineral needs of active folks over 50. As of today, it is unclear what is considered an ideal micronutrient intake for masters athletes. Research on nutritional adequacy of older adults suggest that many fall significantly below the general recommended daily allowance for vitamin A, vitamin D, vitamin E, vitamin C, vitamin B6, folate, thiamine, riboflavin, niacin, and vitamin B12 (Devarshi et al. 2023). Such nutrient deficiencies can compromise overall health and dramatically affect aerobic capacity, muscle strength, power, and endurance.

Not only might we not take in enough of certain micronutrients, those we do take in could be at further risk of deficiencies due to the effects of exercise and aging. Increased urination may lower our vitamin B6 levels, and our body's capacity to synthesize vitamin D decreases with age, possibly requiring supplementation. We also might think megadoses of vitamin C help prevent colds and flu, but its absorption does not slow with age, so an increase may cause kidney impairments, kidney stones, and destruction of vitamin B12. So in this case more is not necessarily better!

Because calcium is a major component of bone, adequate intake is necessary for proper bone growth and maintenance. In response to the epidemic of osteoporosis, the National Academy of Sciences recently boosted calcium recommendations, with 1,000 milligrams now recommended for ages 19 to 50, and 1,200 milligrams for ages 51 and up. Menopausal runners not using hormone replacement may need as much as 1,500 milligrams of calcium each day. To prevent a calcium deficiency, masters athletes should consume three or four servings of dairy each day (e.g., one cup of dairy milk, soy milk, or fortified plant based milks, such as almond or oat, dairy yogurt, or cottage cheese). A calcium supplement, preferably in the citrate or carbonate form, may also be used to boost calcium intake.

Unfortunately, a chronic negative energy balance, common especially among women and those restricting their energy intake, will contribute to lost bone mass, leading to an eight-fold risk for stress fractures. A study of female masters runners discovered an average dietary calcium intake of only 598 milligrams, roughly half the recommended amount (Beshgetoor, Nichols, and Rego 2000), which has been shown to produce calcium stress and lead to an inhibition of bone formation (Åkesson et al. 1998). Weight cycling, as seen in chronic dieters, causes lower spinal and distal radius bone mineral density in women ages 29 to 46 years, exacerbating the risk for osteoporosis especially upon menopause (Fogelholm et al. 1997). All the more reason to get your vitamin D and calcium in your early bone-building years!

But before you rush out and start popping a million different pills every day, take inventory of your food choices and examine where you may be lacking in foods high in specific nutrients. Think leafy greens for vitamin K, lean meats for B vitamins, and dairy products for calcium and vitamin D.

COMMON DRUG–NUTRIENT INTERACTIONS

As we age, it's not uncommon to find ourselves with a growing list of medications to manage various health conditions. While these medications can work wonders for our health, they can also impact how our bodies absorb and use certain nutrients. Let's take a closer look.

Medications such as corticosteroids, used to treat conditions such as arthritis and asthma, can interfere with vitamin D metabolism, potentially leading to lower levels of this crucial nutrient. Considering that vitamin D is essential for bone health, this interaction is particularly important for individuals over 50 who may already be at risk of osteoporosis. Focus on consuming fatty fish (salmon, trout, mackerel); cod liver oil; fortified foods such as fortified dairy products (milk, yogurt, cheese), fortified orange juice, and fortified cereals; and egg yolks.

Blood thinners such as warfarin are often prescribed to prevent blood clots in individuals with conditions such as atrial fibrillation or deep vein thrombosis. However, these medications can interfere with the absorption of vitamin K, which plays a key role in blood clotting. As a result, those on blood thinners should maintain a consistent intake of vitamin K–rich foods to ensure proper clotting function. Focus on consuming leafy greens such as kale, spinach, collard greens, and Swiss chard; broccoli; brussels sprouts; green peas; and soybeans and soy products such as tofu.

Certain medications used to manage acid reflux or ulcers, such as proton pump inhibitors and H2-receptor antagonists, can reduce the absorption of vitamin B12. Since vitamin B12 is crucial for nerve function and red blood cell production, this interaction can lead to symptoms of deficiency, including fatigue and neurological problems, particularly in older adults who may already be at risk of B12 deficiency due to age-related changes in digestion. Focus on consuming animal foods such as beef, pork, poultry, fish, and shellfish; dairy products such as milk, cheese, and yogurt; eggs; and fortified foods such as fortified cereals, fortified plant-based milk alternatives, and nutritional yeast.

Medications such as corticosteroids and certain anticonvulsants can interfere with calcium absorption or increase calcium excretion, putting individuals at risk of bone loss and osteoporosis. It's important for those taking these medications to ensure an adequate intake of calcium through diet or supplementation to support bone health. Focus on consuming dairy products such as milk, cheese, and yogurt; leafy greens such as kale, collard greens, and bok choy; fortified plant-based milk alternatives such as almond milk and soy milk; and canned fish with bones such as sardines and salmon.

Proton pump inhibitors (PPIs), commonly used to treat conditions such as acid reflux and peptic ulcers, can reduce the absorption of iron from food. This can lead to iron-deficiency anemia, characterized by fatigue, weakness, and pale skin. Individuals taking PPIs should monitor their iron levels and consider supplementation if deficiency is detected. Focus on consuming red meat such as beef, lamb, and liver; poultry such as chicken and turkey; fish and shellfish; legumes such as lentils, chickpeas, and beans; and iron-fortified cereals and breads.

PPIs can also interfere with the absorption of zinc, an essential mineral involved in immune function, wound healing, and metabolism. Zinc deficiency can impair immune function and lead to a variety of health issues, so it's important for individuals taking PPIs to ensure an adequate intake of zinc through diet or supplementation. Focus on consuming shellfish such as oysters, crab, and lobster; red meat such as beef and lamb; poultry such as chicken and turkey; dairy products such as milk, cheese, and yogurt; legumes such as chickpeas, lentils, and beans; and nuts and seeds such as pumpkin seeds, cashews, and almonds.

Understanding and managing drug–nutrient interactions is essential for individuals over 50 who may be taking multiple medications. By being aware of these interactions and taking steps to mitigate their impact, such as adjusting dietary intake or considering supplementation, individuals can optimize their nutritional status and overall health as they continue their strength-training journey.

SPORT SUPPLEMENTS

Ah, sport supplements, the secret sauce that can take your workouts from meh to magnificent. Just do a search for "sport supplements" and see how many hits come up! Yes, it's overwhelming, and with so many options, it can be hard to know which ones are worth your hard-earned cash and which have credible research behind them. Even when macronutrient (carbs, protein, and fat) and total energy (calorie) requirements are met, some micronutrient supplements may still be needed. The requirements are based on current research to help support masters athletes better retain muscle mass and combat the age-related muscle loss. As the evidence evolves, so may the recommendations! If in doubt always consult a registered sports dietitian to get the most up to date information.

Let's start by looking at one of the most popular supplements: protein powder.

Protein Powder

As mentioned in the macronutrient section of this chapter, protein requirements for individuals over 50 who are strength training are higher compared to sedentary adults because muscle protein synthesis tends to be less efficient with age and depends on factors such as activity level, muscle mass, and overall health status. If meeting these protein needs and timing through whole foods is challenging, or if you have increased protein requirements due to intense training or specific health conditions, protein supplements may help bridge the gap.

A well-balanced diet rich in lean meats, poultry, fish, dairy, eggs, legumes, nuts, and seeds can provide all the protein and essential amino acids needed for muscle repair and growth. However, if you choose to opt out of dairy foods or are enjoying more vegan styles of eating, it may be more challenging for you to meet your needs through foods alone.

Supplements can be a convenient and portable option for getting a quick dose of protein, especially after workouts when whole food options may be less convenient. They can also be helpful for those with busy lifestyles or who struggle to consume enough protein from whole foods alone. If your goal is to optimize muscle growth, recovery, and overall performance, supplements may provide a convenient and efficient way to increase protein intake and support these goals. But which ones to choose?

When choosing a protein supplement, consider factors such as your dietary preferences, nutritional needs, and fitness goals to determine which type is best suited for you. It's also essential to select high-quality products from reputable brands to ensure safety and efficacy.

Let's break down the various types.

Whey Protein

Whey protein is derived from milk and is one of the most popular and widely available protein supplements. It is rich in essential amino acids, particularly branched-chain amino acids, and has a high biological value, meaning it is efficiently used by the body for muscle repair and growth. Branched-chain amino acids (BCAAs)—leucine, isoleucine, and valine—are important for recovery from exercise because they play critical roles in muscle protein synthesis and reducing muscle damage and soreness. Whole foods rich in BCAAs (like whey, dairy, eggs, meat, and soy) are more effective than isolated BCAAs because they provide all essential amino acids needed for full muscle repair. Whey protein is often favored for its rapid digestion and absorption, making it an ideal choice for post-workout recovery.

Types of whey protein include whey protein concentrate, whey protein isolate, and whey protein hydrolysate. Whey protein concentrate contains varying amounts of protein (usually around 70 to 80 percent) along with some carbohydrates and fats. Whey protein isolate contains a higher percentage of protein (typically 90 percent or higher) and minimal amounts of carbohydrates and fats. Whey protein hydrolysate is a predigested form of whey protein, which may be easier for some to digest and absorb.

Casein Protein

Like whey, casein protein is also derived from milk but is digested and absorbed more slowly. It forms a gel-like substance in the stomach, which slows digestion and provides a steady release of amino acids into the bloodstream over several hours. This makes it a suitable option for nighttime use or for individuals looking for prolonged muscle protein synthesis and satiety.

The types of casein protein are casein protein concentrate and casein protein isolate. Casein protein concentrate contains around 70 to 80 percent protein, along with some carbohydrates and fats. Casein protein isolate contains a higher percentage of protein (usually around 90 percent) and minimal amounts of carbohydrates and fats.

Soy Protein

Soy protein is derived from soybeans and is a popular plant-based protein supplement. It is a complete protein source, meaning it contains all essential amino acids. It is also rich in fiber, vitamins, and minerals. Soy protein has been shown to have various health benefits, including supporting heart health and reducing cholesterol levels.

Soy protein is available as soy protein isolate, which contains around 90 percent protein and minimal amounts of carbohydrates and fats.

Pea Protein

Pea protein is derived from yellow split peas and is another popular plant-based protein supplement. It is rich in branched-chain amino acids, but it isn't considered a complete protein source, meaning that it is lacking in one or more of the essential amino acids and is also low in the all-star amino acid leucine.

Pea protein is available as pea protein isolate, which contains around 85 to 90 percent protein and minimal amounts of carbohydrates and fats.

Rice Protein

Rice protein is derived from brown rice and is similar to other plant-based protein supplements (except soy) in that while it is not a complete protein source on its own, it can be combined with other plant-based protein sources to form a complete amino-acid profile.

Rice protein is available as rice protein concentrate or rice protein isolate. Rice protein concentrate contains around 70 to 80 percent protein, along with some carbohydrates and fats. Rice protein isolate contains a higher percentage of protein (usually around 90 percent) and minimal amounts of carbohydrates and fats.

Selecting a Quality Supplement

Navigating the endless sea of sport supplements can be daunting and confusing. Choosing the right supplement is especially important to support individual performance, recovery, and overall health goals while minimizing risks. Here are a few tips to consider when diving into the supplement sea to keep you supplement savvy.

- Look for supplements that have undergone independent third-party testing to ensure they are free from banned substances. Reliable third-party certifications include NSF Certified for Sport, Informed Sport, and BSCG (Banned Substances Control Group). These certifications help minimize the risk of unintentional doping violations.

- Check the supplement facts label (USA and other regions) and ingredients list. Look for transparency—avoid proprietary blends that don't disclose exact ingredient amounts. Choose high-quality, evidence-based ingredients and avoid excessive additives, artificial sweeteners, or fillers. Verify the supplement facts table to understand what's in the product. Pay attention to serving size, active ingredients, and dosages.

- Know what you are taking and why. Be clear on the purpose of the supplement and whether it aligns with your specific needs (e.g., performance, recovery, hydration). Check for credible scientific evidence supporting the effectiveness of the supplement for your goals.

- Avoid red flags. I like to call this "Be Nutrition-Quackery Savvy." Be cautious of products that make unsupported, exaggerated claims ("Build muscle overnight!"), use proprietary blends without disclosing ingredient amounts, lack third-party testing or Good Manufacturing Practices certification, or are endorsed by famous people without supporting evidence.

- Consult a sports dietitian. A sports dietitian can help assess whether a supplement is necessary and recommend evidence-based choices.

If it sounds too good to be true, then it probably is!

Creatine

This bad boy has been a long-standing supplement and is well researched in all age groups. It's been gaining more and more support to help improve strength and power and improve the anaerobic energy source ATP (adenosine triphosphate) during bouts of intermittent, high-intensity exercise. There is a growing body of evidence showing that creatine supplementation, particularly when combined with exercise, provides musculoskeletal and performance benefits in older adults (Candow et al. 2022). It has also been shown to help speed up recovery after exercise-induced muscle damage (Wax et al. 2021). Research suggests that older athletes may see increased muscle mass gain and strength from the addition of creatine monohydrate to resistance training (Tarnopolsky et al. 2007). There is, however, limited data for athletes over the age of 70. Masters athletes with kidney problems should discuss the use of creatine with their general practitioner or sport physician.

To increase your creatine stores, you can safely take 3 to 5 grams per day for 4 to 6 weeks (or longer) with a good source of carbohydrates and protein; I usually recommend taking it in the postrecovery snack since it is most practical and will give adequate carbohydrates. This can help with improving strength and fat-free mass. Especially if you are vegan, supplementing may provide significant increases in intramuscular creatine.

Omega-3

The benefits of omega-3s were discussed in the fats section of this chapter. In addition, a few studies have reported that fish oil supplementation (2 to 4 grams per day taken when most convenient) could increase muscle anabolic response to resistance training and adequate protein intake in adults of all ages associated with gains in strength and functional capacity (Heileson et al. 2023). If you find it difficult to get in good sources of omega-3 (approximately 3 to 4 servings [3 ounces] of fatty fish per week) then you may benefit from a supplement.

Caffeine

Ah, caffeine, the ultimate pick-me-up for those early morning workouts. As for caffeine supplements to help with strength training in athletes over 50, it's important to approach caffeine consumption with caution and consider individual factors such as sensitivity to caffeine, overall health status, and preexisting medical conditions. While caffeine can provide benefits such as increased alertness, improved focus, and enhanced performance (reducing time to fatigue) during workouts, excessive caffeine intake can lead to negative side effects such as jitteriness, increased heart rate, and disrupted sleep.

Here are some general recommendations for caffeine intake:

- **Start with a low dose.** If you're not accustomed to caffeine or have sensitivity to it, start with a low dose and gradually increase as tolerated (2 to 3 milligrams per kilogram of body weight working up to 5 milligrams per kilogram of body weight as tolerated).
- **Time it right.** Try to consume caffeine 30 to 60 minutes before your strength-training session to maximize its effects, but one size doesn't fit all here. We metabolize caffeine according to our genes, so what works for one may not work for others.

- **Stay hydrated.** Caffeine has diuretic effects, so be sure to drink plenty of water throughout the day to stay hydrated, especially if you're consuming caffeine before exercise.
- **Avoid excess caffeine.** Be mindful of your total caffeine intake from all sources, including coffee, tea, energy drinks, and caffeine-containing supplements.

It's always a good idea to consult with a healthcare professional or registered dietitian before starting any new supplement regimen, including caffeine supplements, especially if you have underlying health conditions or are taking medications that may interact with caffeine.

Beetroot

Beetroot supplementation, particularly in the form of nitrate-rich beetroot juice, has gained attention for its potential benefits for athletes, including individuals over 50 who engage in strength training. Benefits include improved exercise performance, increased muscle efficiency, and potentially reduced oxygen cost of exercise (Domínguex et al. 2017). However, individual responses may vary, and more research is needed to fully understand the long-term effects and optimal dosing strategies for beet supplementation.

As always, it's essential to consult with a healthcare professional before starting any new supplement regimen, especially if you have underlying health conditions or are taking medications. So before you go and "just beet it" (I know you '80s folks will get that!), let's delve a bit deeper into the potential benefits to sports performance and training with beet supplementation.

Beetroot may improve exercise performance. Nitrate, found abundantly in beets and beetroot juice, is converted into nitric oxide in the body. Nitric oxide plays a crucial role in vasodilation (widening of blood vessels), and this dilation may enhance blood flow and oxygen delivery to muscles during exercise, potentially improving exercise performance, endurance, and recovery.

Beetroot may increase muscle efficiency. Nitric oxide may also improve muscle efficiency by enhancing mitochondrial function, which is responsible for energy production within muscle cells. This increased efficiency can potentially lead to improved muscle function and endurance during strength-training sessions.

Some research suggests that beet supplementation may reduce the oxygen cost of exercise, meaning that individuals may require less oxygen to perform the same amount of work. This can be particularly beneficial for older adults, as it may improve exercise tolerance and reduce fatigue during strength-training sessions.

Beetroot supplementation has potential benefits for blood pressure. Nitric oxide's role in vasodilation may help lower blood pressure, which could be particularly beneficial for older adults at increased risk of hypertension. However, individuals with existing low blood pressure should exercise caution with beet supplementation, as it may further lower blood pressure to undesirable levels.

Here are considerations for beet supplementation:

- **Dosage:** Research studies have used varying dosages of beetroot juice, typically ranging from 300 to 500 milliliters per day. It's essential to follow dosage recommendations provided by reputable sources or consult with a healthcare professional before starting beet supplementation.
- **Timing:** Consuming beetroot juice 2 to 3 hours before exercise has been shown effective in enhancing exercise performance. However, individual

responses may vary, so experimenting with timing may be necessary to determine what works best for you.

- **Side effects:** Beet supplementation is generally safe for most individuals when consumed in moderation. However, some people may experience gastrointestinal discomfort or changes in urine color (due to the presence of betalain pigments). If you experience adverse effects, discontinue use and consult with a healthcare professional.

Collagen

Last but not least, let's talk collagen. It's a popular one for sure, especially in the older age category. More research is needed to fully understand the effects of collagen supplementation on strength-training outcomes, but let's take a look at each potential benefit and you can be your own judge.

Collagen supplementation may support joint health. Collagen is a structural protein found in connective tissues throughout the body, including joints, tendons, ligaments, and cartilage. As we age, collagen production naturally declines, which can contribute to joint stiffness, discomfort, and reduced mobility. Collagen supplementation may help support joint health by providing the building blocks needed for the maintenance and repair of connective tissues.

Collagen may help muscle recovery and repair. In addition to its role in joint health, collagen is also a key component of muscle tissue. Some research suggests that collagen supplementation may help support muscle recovery and repair following strength-training sessions. Collagen contains specific amino acids, such as glycine, proline, and hydroxyproline, which are essential for muscle protein synthesis and repair.

Here are considerations for collagen supplementation:

- **Type of collagen:** Collagen supplements are available in various forms, including hydrolyzed collagen peptides, collagen protein powders, and collagen-containing foods and beverages. Hydrolyzed collagen peptides are broken down into smaller, more easily absorbed fragments, making them a popular choice for supplementation. Remember that you can also make your own—bone broth is a great source of collagen!

- **Dosage:** Dosage recommendations for collagen supplementation vary depending on the specific product and intended use. Studies have used dosages ranging from 2.5 to 15 grams of collagen peptides per day for improving connective tissue and muscle recovery. It's essential to follow dosage recommendations provided by reputable sources or consult with a healthcare professional for personalized advice.

- **Timing:** Collagen supplementation can be consumed at any time of day, with or without food. Some individuals prefer to take collagen supplements in the morning or before bed, while others may incorporate them into postworkout shakes or smoothies for muscle recovery.

WRAPPING UP

And there you have it—everything you need to know about fueling your strength-training journey over 50. Remember, nutrition is just one piece of the puzzle, but it's a darn important one. So, fuel your body with the good stuff, listen to what it's telling you, and get ready to crush those workouts like never before. You've got this!

CHAPTER 4

Assessments

Now that we know just how important proper strength training and nutrition are for strong, robust aging, the question becomes "Where do we begin?"

This may surprise you, but I don't use fitness assessments aside from a physical activity readiness questionnaire. Perhaps I'm still scarred from the President's Council on Physical Fitness test from grade school, every Gen-X kid's first physical assessment. Do you remember the miserable gauntlet of push-ups, pull-ups (boys) or flexed arm hang (girls), sit-ups, sit and reach, shuttle run, and mile run? It was a test I could never quite pass to earn that crappy patch I wanted so badly.

In my programs the first few workouts *are* the assessment, as I prefer to see how a client performs doing the actual exercises in their program rather than make them do an arbitrary movement screen that may have little bearing on where I start them.

One exercise used in some screenings is the overhead squat, but in training clients over 32 years, I've *never* started with an overhead squat. In fact, very few clients have ever done one at all, even after decades training with me. This doesn't mean the overhead squat is a bad exercise, but I consider it a highly technical, advanced exercise that most people never need to do. So rather than testing the overhead squat, I'll assess a client with less advanced exercises such as the goblet squat and overhead press. We'll use these in their program, and they'll give me similar insights into their form and current capabilities with fewer risks.

GENERAL HEALTH ASSESSMENT

I know you're reading this book to learn to get stronger, but over 50, your goal should also be to be as healthy as possible. And the best way to assess the current state of your health is to get your physical and blood work done. Even those who appear lean and fit on the outside can have the beginnings of heart disease, diabetes, nonalcoholic fatty liver disease, and more.

Why did I include this in a book about strength training? Because I recently had my own health scare after routine blood work, which proved to be the wake-up call I didn't know I needed. It had been about two years since my last blood test (my mistake!), although all prior blood work had been great, even into my 50s. But in the two years since that blood work, I'd gained about 30 pounds (not all muscle), and was back up to the highest weight of my life (nearly 220 pounds).

Luckily for me, we have a urologist client at my gym, and he encouraged me to come in and get my PSA (prostate-specific antigen) levels checked since I hadn't had it tested in two years, and the values, although still normal, had been slowly rising over the prior seven years. Shockingly, my PSA levels were actually better than when first tested! Fortunately, he also did a comprehensive metabolic panel and A1C test. The results floored me. They showed I was diabetic *and* had nonalcoholic fatty liver disease!

Diabetes?! Fatty liver?! But I felt fine, and I was strong as ever in the gym—heck, I could bench press 300 pounds. Yes, I was a little overweight, but I was far from obese. How could this happen to *me*? In hindsight, I should have known better. For months prior to those blood tests, I had been eating with reckless abandon: pizza, ice cream, burgers, fries, Thai food, anything. Food delivery was my friend.

To make matters worse, I had also been far less regular with my strength training, going from four days a week the first half of the year to once or twice *a month* by year's end. I wasn't even reaching my goal of 8,000 steps most days, let alone doing any real cardio. For months I had been both incredibly sedentary and eating extremely poorly. Adding to my misery, I also had my first bout with COVID…an unhealthy time to say the least.

Normally you wouldn't expect a few months of poor choices to have such a dramatic impact on your health, but it did. We still aren't sure why. I never knew my father, so perhaps I have a genetic predisposition to diabetes or fatty liver that I had kept at bay by making better choices. All I can say is that I was lucky to catch this stuff early and that I'm able to use my knowledge of diet and exercise to reverse the damage.

I mentioned in the introduction that my goal is to remove the impediments that block people from strength training, so unless you currently suffer from a medical condition or injury that requires a doctor's care, you don't have to wait for an annual physical or blood work to start training. But please consider doing so sooner rather than later, especially if it's been a while since your last physical. I'll climb down off my soapbox now.

MATCH ASSESSMENTS TO YOUR GOALS

I don't find most of the fitness assessments commonly used in a gym setting to be particularly useful. They often do little more than score your ability to perform a specific test, and they tend to label people by their dysfunctions, according to each test's scoring system. What could be more depressing than finally committing to go to the gym and get in shape, only to have the trainer tell you how dysfunctional you are? "Thanks, Chase, I think I'll just go home and eat a pint of ice cream now."

Does this mean all assessments are unnecessary and aren't beneficial? No. However, the assessment you use should matter to *you*. If your goal is to lose body fat, test your percent body fat (and your scale weight) to determine your current condition. You can retest later to assess the effectiveness of your strength training and nutrition program. But again, don't let the lack of a body-fat test stop you from starting training. Millions of people have trained and lost body fat without having their fat pinched (skinfold test), being hydrostatically (underwater) weighed, or having a DEXA (dual X-ray absorptiometry) scan. The mirror and how your clothes fit may be all the assessment you need.

Similarly, if you've been told you need to improve your blood pressure or resting heart rate, it's a good idea to know these values before you start training. But again, lack of these tests shouldn't keep you from starting. Special note: If you have or suspect you have existing cardiac issues or have a family history, I encourage you to wear a heart rate monitor during exercise.

Many trainers require clients to take "before" pictures and circumference measurements, which can be terrifying for prospective trainees, so I don't take them unless asked. Progress pictures can be motivating for some trainees, but others may find them demotivating because change happens slowly and gradually, with no dramatic "before and after" transformation common in fitness marketing. Be patient with yourself and wait a few months before taking "after" pictures. If you can wait, in time you'll probably be glad you did take "before" pictures. Even if you don't take official pictures, I'm sure you have casual photos you are unhappy with that would suffice.

STRENGTH ASSESSMENTS

I have a similar opinion on strength testing. Some coaches use max testing to gauge the current absolute strength level of a new client. I don't find that necessary. And the few clients I work with who are competitive powerlifters already know their maxes, so I don't even need to test them.

I prefer to think of assessments as an ongoing awareness of how your body feels on a given day, not a random test performed at irregular intervals. Each training session, the first questions I ask every client are "How are you feeling today?" and "Does anything feel sore or out of sorts since the last workout?" That's really the only preworkout assessment I need. Those who are training on their own should do a self-assessment and adjust that day's training plan as needed.

Every rep of every set of every workout is an assessment, but only of your ability on *that* day. There are simply too many variables that can affect the performance of the average trainee from day to day. Lack of sleep, home or work stress, poor nutrition, or overindulgence in alcohol can all impact how you feel and what you can accomplish within a workout.

The main reason I don't find max testing to be necessary is that I intentionally start every new client out with very light weights. So light, in fact, that they can usually perform three sets of 12 to 15 reps in good form (as you'll see in the beginner program in chapter 11). I do this for a few reasons. First, a client may have a joint or muscle issue they mentioned on their intake form. And even though I choose exercises I don't think will aggravate their condition, you never know, so I'd rather find out about an issue while using a lighter weight than one closer to their current maximum.

Also, people often forget about things like the ankle they sprained playing soccer in college but never finished rehabbing. Even though they don't think about that long-ago injury, their lack of range of motion at the ankle will show up on an exercise like the step-up or a squat. I could spend the first session testing their ankle range of motion with a goniometer, but it won't give me any better insight into their abilities than a set of step-ups, so I'd rather get to training and see what happens than spend our limited time measuring joint angles.

Simply put, the process of training will naturally improve strength, mobility, balance, and coordination. I focus on improvements from workout to workout using exercises that are in my programs, rather than arbitrary strength testing or fancy movement screens.

My opinion on assessments was solidified after I asked an esteemed colleague with a PhD in nutrition if they recommended their clients get specific blood work done to determine vitamin and mineral deficiencies before starting them on a nutrition program. His response surprised me. He said, "No. I don't recommend testing because it isn't going to affect the recommendations of the program, so why put the client through it?"

His point was that even if someone was deficient in a specific nutrient, it wasn't going to change the recommendation to eat a varied diet of more fruits, vegetables, legumes, and dairy, which would already address said deficiency. By not requiring blood work, he removed an obstacle he felt was unnecessary and might prevent clients from starting to change their dietary habits. This made so much sense to me, and it changed some of my opinions of movement screens, strength testing, and what is truly necessary for an initial assessment.

ASSESSING SHOULDER FLEXION

So are there *any* fitness assessments I require when beginning training? Really only one: the shoulder flexion test. Before I have someone overhead press, I need to know their ability to fully flex the shoulder; in other words, can they lift their arms straight overhead without arching their lower back to compensate?

This test can be performed standing or lying on a mat. I have clients do it standing because I can correct them if they are arching their low back to compensate, and it more closely mimics the exercises we'll be doing. However, if you are training solo and want to make sure you don't cheat, simply lie on the floor on a mat.

Whether standing up or lying on a mat, raise both arms together, starting at your sides and finishing as close to overhead as possible. Ideally, the arms should be in line with the ears at the top. Many people don't have the shoulder mobility to do this at all, or at least not without arching their lower back and raising their chest excessively (called rib flare).

Figures 4.1 and 4.2 show the shoulder flexion test from lying and standing positions.

If you are unable to fully flex the shoulder, I would not start out with dumbbell or barbell overhead presses but instead would use a landmine apparatus (if available) or you can wedge one end of a barbell into a corner or against something stable to mimic the landmine. See chapter 7 for all landmine pressing options.

Other than the shoulder flexion test (which I do on day two of my assessment workout), most trainees should be able to jump right into the training programs in this book. Also, if you've had a bit of a layoff since training with weights, don't feel like you need to "get in shape" *before* strength training. While good cardiovascular conditioning is important and something you can develop concurrently with weight training, there are no conditioning prerequisites for strength training.

And remember, each workout is an assessment of how you are feeling that day and how you performed compared to prior workouts. Strive to use more weight or do more reps or use even better form. Keep a workout journal and refer to it often. Make notes of anything like illness, injuries, or poor sleep that may have caused you to not do as well on an exercise as the last time, but realize that in

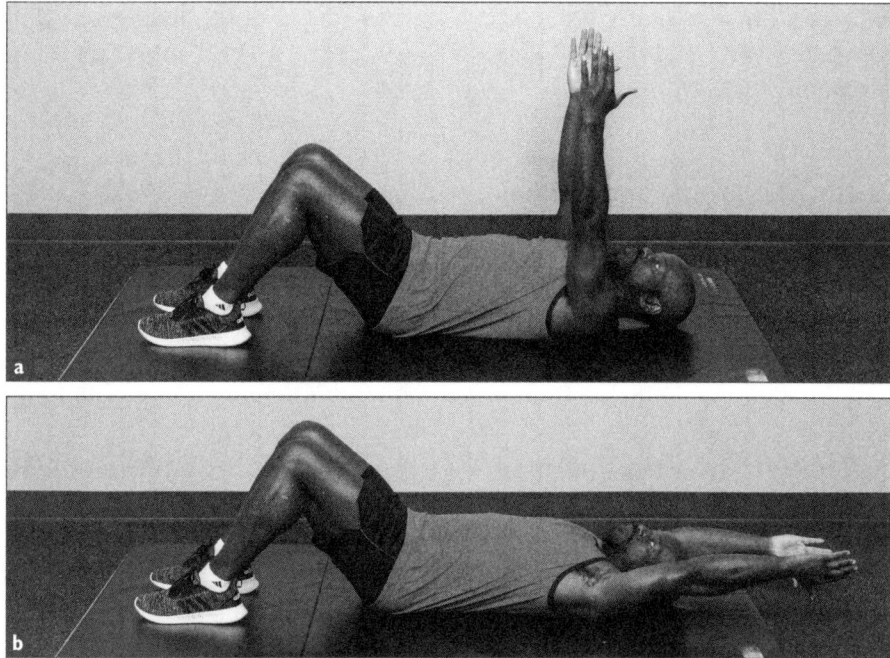

FIGURE 4.1 Shoulder flexion test from lying position: *(a)* starting position and *(b)* reaching arms overhead.

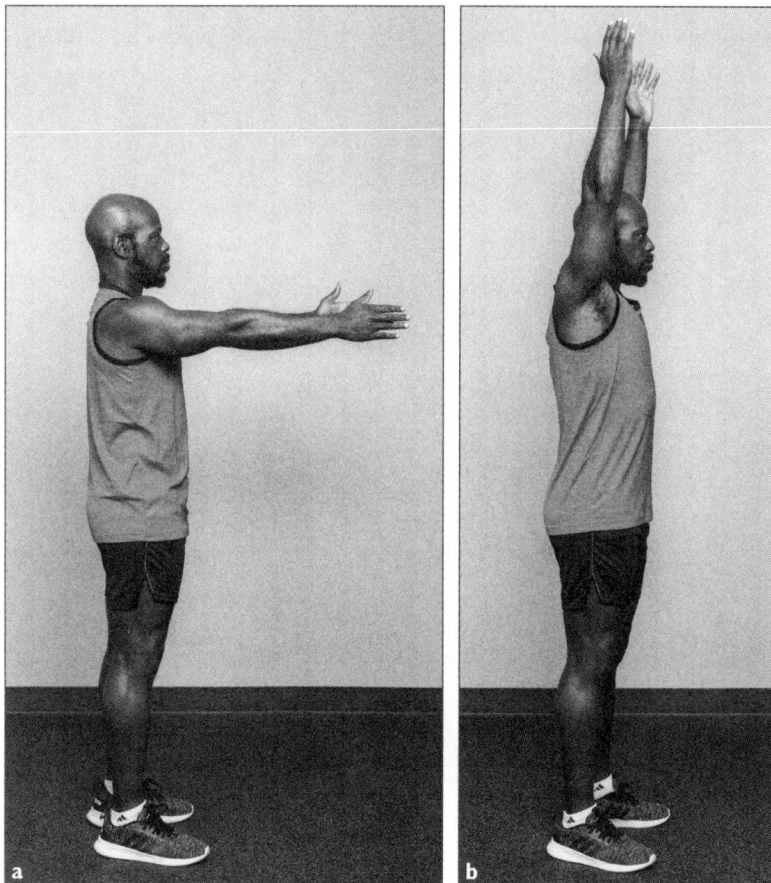

FIGURE 4.2 Shoulder flexion test from standing position: *(a)* starting position and *(b)* reaching arms overhead.

our 50s, we'll have as many workouts where we fight not to lose ground as we do hitting new personal records, and that's OK! Let's go to the next chapter and dig into some actual training!

CHAPTER 5

Warm-Up

Warm-ups have come a long way since I played high school sports in the 1980s. Back then a warm-up usually consisted of a couple of light stretches, some bouncing around on the toes, and then a run—always a run. Oh, how times have changed!

These days, it's not uncommon to see recommendations to do a general warm-up, then mobility work, some foam rolling, and a few activation drills, and then, *if* you have any time left, you can do your workout. I'm exhausted just thinking about it. Is that much warm-up necessary?

While there is no one-size-fits-all recommendation, not warming up could leave you susceptible to injury, but overdoing it can sap the time and energy needed for strength training itself. A meta-analysis of 32 trials showed that 79 percent of the studies reported a performance benefit when an appropriate warm-up was done beforehand (Fradkin, Zazryn, and Smoliga 2010). However, this wasn't proven true in every study, but when the researchers dug into those studies, they speculated that the type of warm-up used wasn't specific to the activities that followed.

What we do know is this: A dynamic warm-up where we move the body similarly to the training that follows gets better results than old-school passive methods of static stretching or a sauna, for example. Think about warming up like blowing into an old Nintendo cartridge before playing Mario—a short ritual to ensure the real action runs glitch-free!

Based on the following potential benefits, at least *some* warm-up is a good idea:

- **Increased body temperature:** A rise in core and muscle temperature makes muscle fibers more pliable and efficient (Bishop 2003).

- **Improved blood circulation:** Elevating the heart rate increases blood flow to the muscles, ensuring they are sufficiently supplied with oxygen and nutrients (McGowan et al. 2015).

- **Enhanced muscle performance:** Adequately warmed muscles contract more forcefully, relax more quickly, and allow a greater range of motion (Fradkin, Zazryn, and Smoliga 2010; Stewart and Sleivert 1998).

- **Injury prevention:** By gradually increasing the demands on your musculoskeletal system, you reduce the risk of strains, sprains, and other injuries (Shellock and Prentice 1985).

- **Mental preparation:** The warm-up provides a brief window to focus on technique and establish mind-muscle connection before the main sets (McGowan et al. 2015).
- **Hormone production:** The warm-up can help stimulate the body's release of hormones responsible for regulating energy production (Bishop 2003).
- **Joint lubrication:** The warm-up circulates synovial fluid, reducing the friction between joints and improving their mobility (Shellock and Prentice 1985).

PERSONALIZE THE WARM-UP

My recommendation on the warm-up is the same as my advice on training: Aim for the minimum effective dose to get the job done, then move on. Some people require very little warm-up, and others need more. Do as much or as little as you need on a given day based on how your body feels and what the workout entails.

At minimum, I recommend 3 to 5 minutes of general warm-up to elevate the heart rate, get a little sweat going, and create a mental buffer between the outside world and the gym. I've found it's just as important to leave the stress of the day outside as it is to warm up the tissues of the body.

I prefer warm-ups that include both the upper and lower body muscles; an elliptical machine or the Schwinn Airdyne (fan bike) work well here. However, if you prefer to warm up on the treadmill or recumbent bike, that's fine too. If using a more intense warm-up like the fan bike, just 2 to 3 minutes may get the job done (and surprisingly well for such a short duration!), while 5 to 10 minutes may be necessary for less intense activities such as treadmill walking.

Jumping rope is a great total body warm-up that's also convenient, portable, and low cost. However, use caution: Older bodies tend to be stiffer, and doing ballistic, plyometric exercises (bouncing or jumping) when the body isn't already warmed up could be a bit risky. But if you like jumping rope and can do it pain-free, it does provide a thorough warm-up in a short time.

Many trainees will be able to go directly into lifting after a short general warm-up. Others, especially those with hip or shoulder issues, may need a more thorough, specific warm-up before weight training. For those who do need a bit more warm-up, I recommend the following mobility work for the hips and shoulders:

Shoulder Warm-Up

1. Arm circle (figure 5.1): Stand tall with your arms extended to the sides at shoulder height. Perform small circles forward for 20 to 30 seconds, gradually increasing the diameter. Reverse the direction and repeat for the same duration. Keep your shoulders relaxed and avoid shrugging.
2. Scapular wall slide (figure 5.2): Stand with your back against a wall, arms bent in a goalpost or W shape, with wrists, elbows, and shoulders touching the wall. Slide your arms upward while maintaining contact with the wall. Slowly return to the starting position. Focus on controlled movement and scapular engagement.
3. Band pull-apart (figure 5.3): Hold a resistance band with both hands at shoulder height, arms extended. Pull the band apart by moving your arms outward, squeezing the shoulder blades together. Pause briefly, then return to the start with control. Keep your arms straight and your shoulders down throughout.

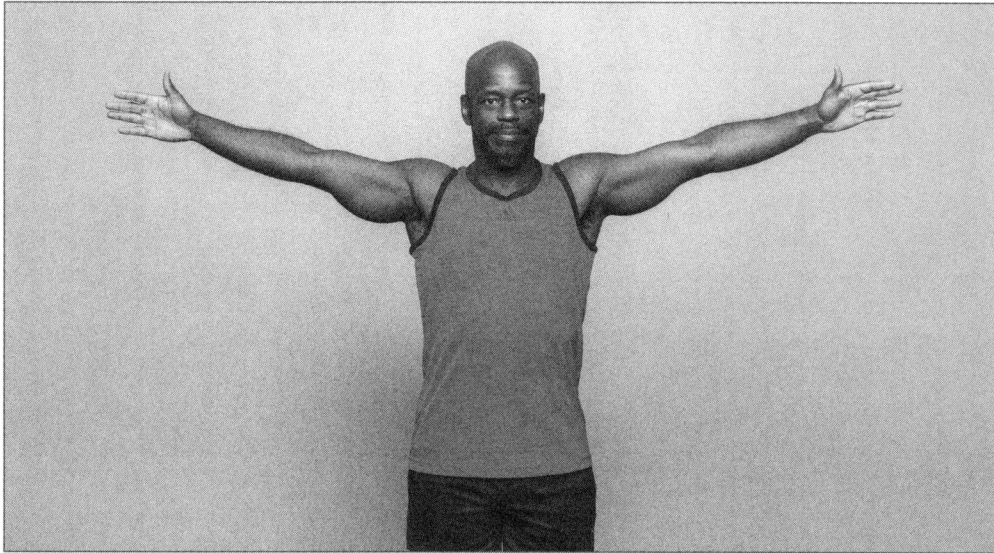

FIGURE 5.1   Shoulder warm-up: arm circle.

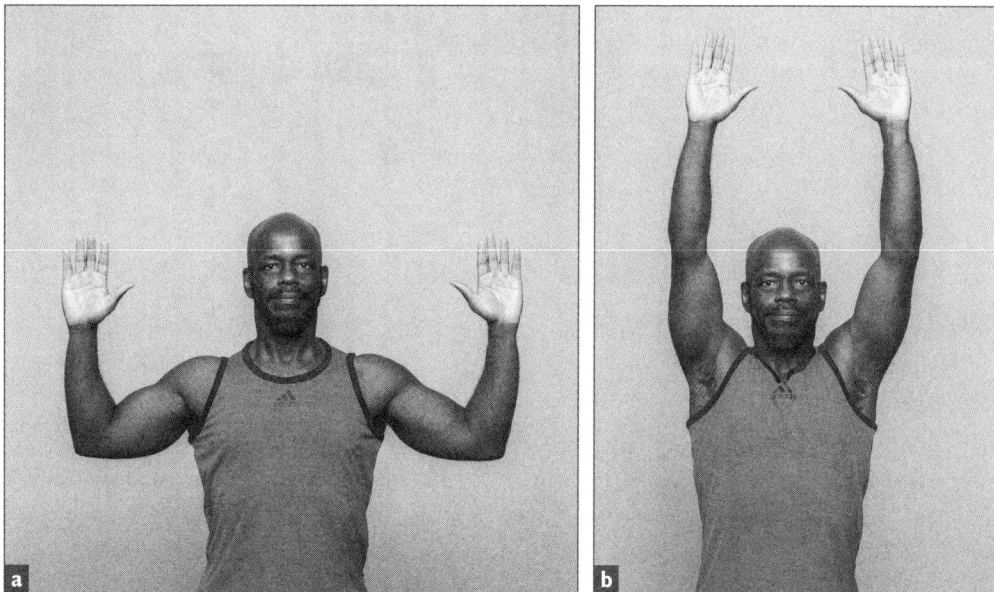

FIGURE 5.2   Shoulder warm-up: scapular wall slide.

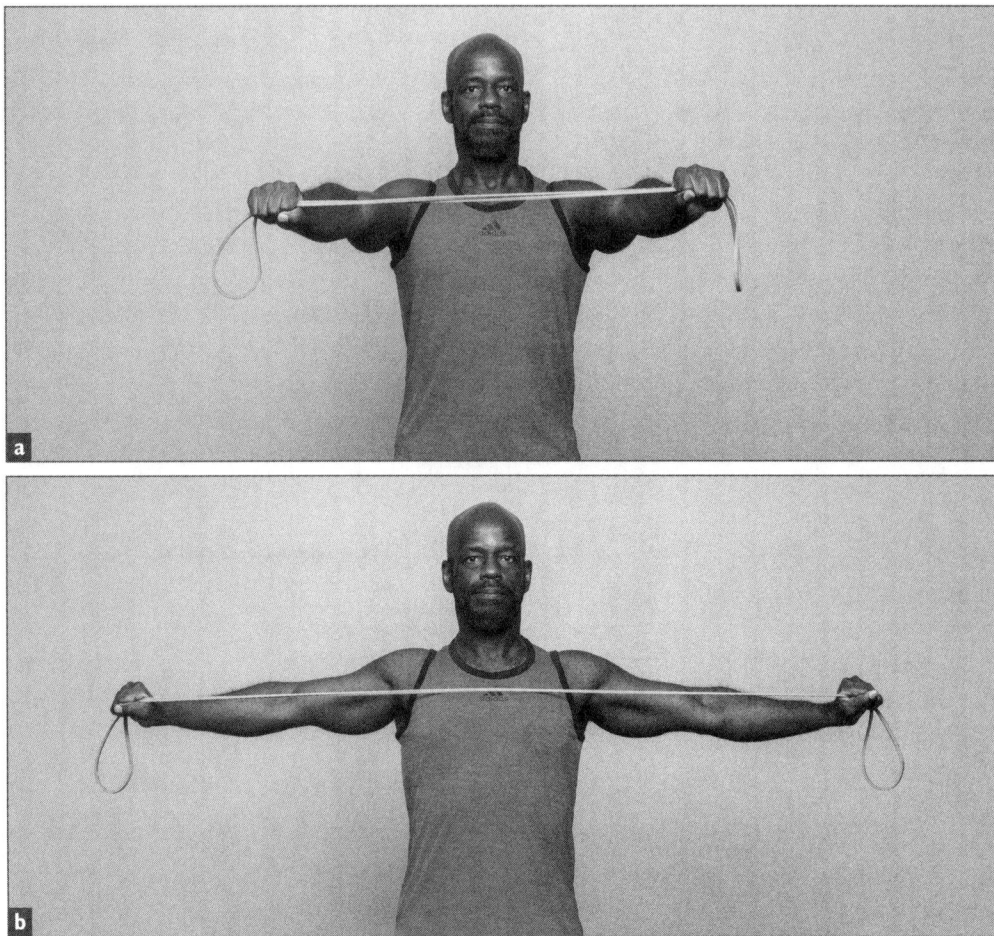

FIGURE 5.3 Shoulder warm-up: band pull-apart.

Hip Warm-Up

1. Hip circle (figure 5.4): Kneel on all fours. Lift one knee out to the side (about 90 degrees) and draw slow, controlled circles with your knee. Perform 5 to 10 circles clockwise and counterclockwise, then switch legs. Keep your core engaged and your spine neutral.

2. Leg swing (figure 5.5): Hold onto a wall or post for balance if needed. You may want to stand on a low step or box so the leg can swing freely without hitting the ground. Swing one leg forward and backward in a controlled motion (10 to 15 reps). Then swing it side to side across your body (10 to 15 reps). Repeat with the other leg. Keep your upper body tall and your movement smooth.

3. World's greatest stretch (figure 5.6): Step into a deep lunge with your back leg extended and both hands on the floor inside the front foot. Rotate your upper body toward the front leg, reaching that arm toward the ceiling. Hold briefly, then return to the floor and switch sides. This opens up the hips, thoracic spine, and hamstrings in one movement.

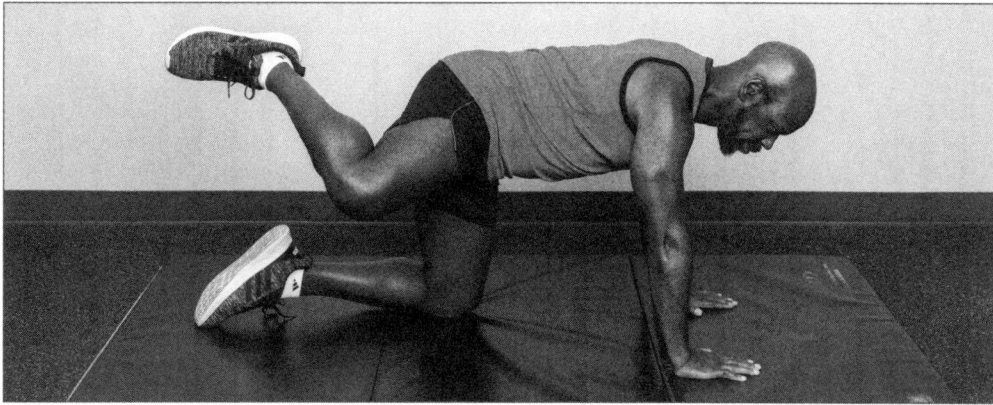

FIGURE 5.4 Hip warm-up: hip circle.

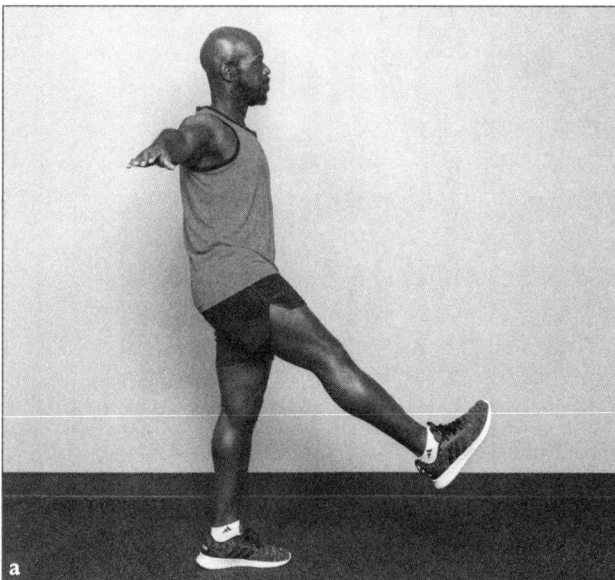

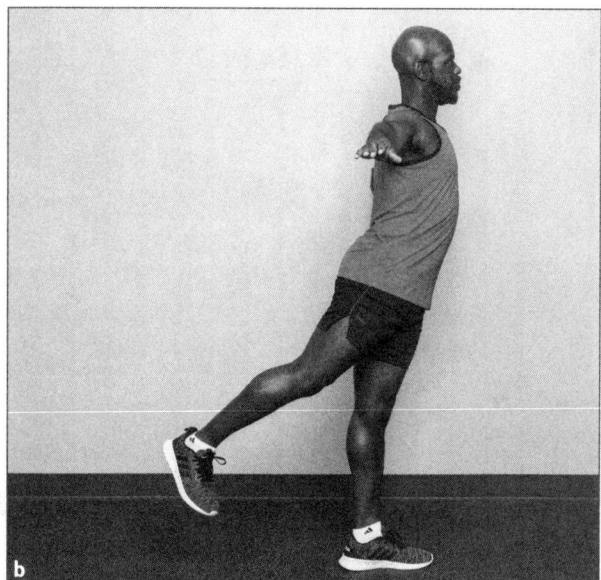

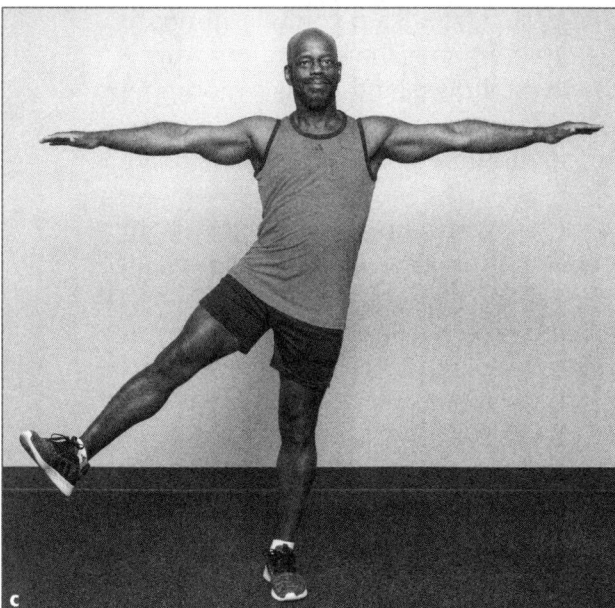

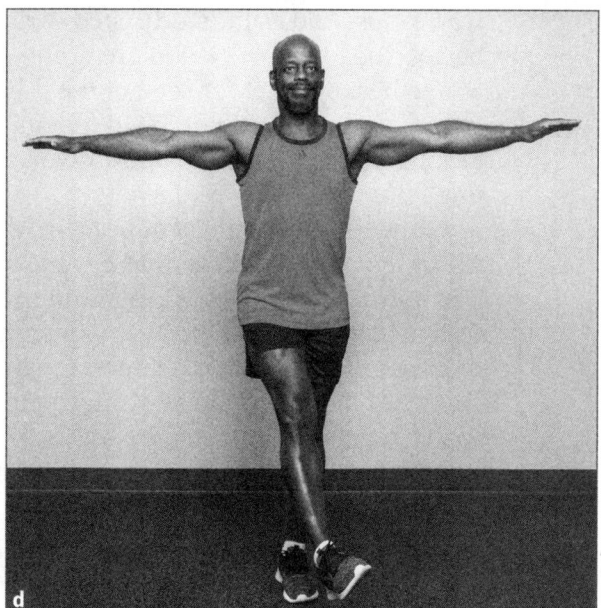

FIGURE 5.5 Hip warm-up: leg swing.

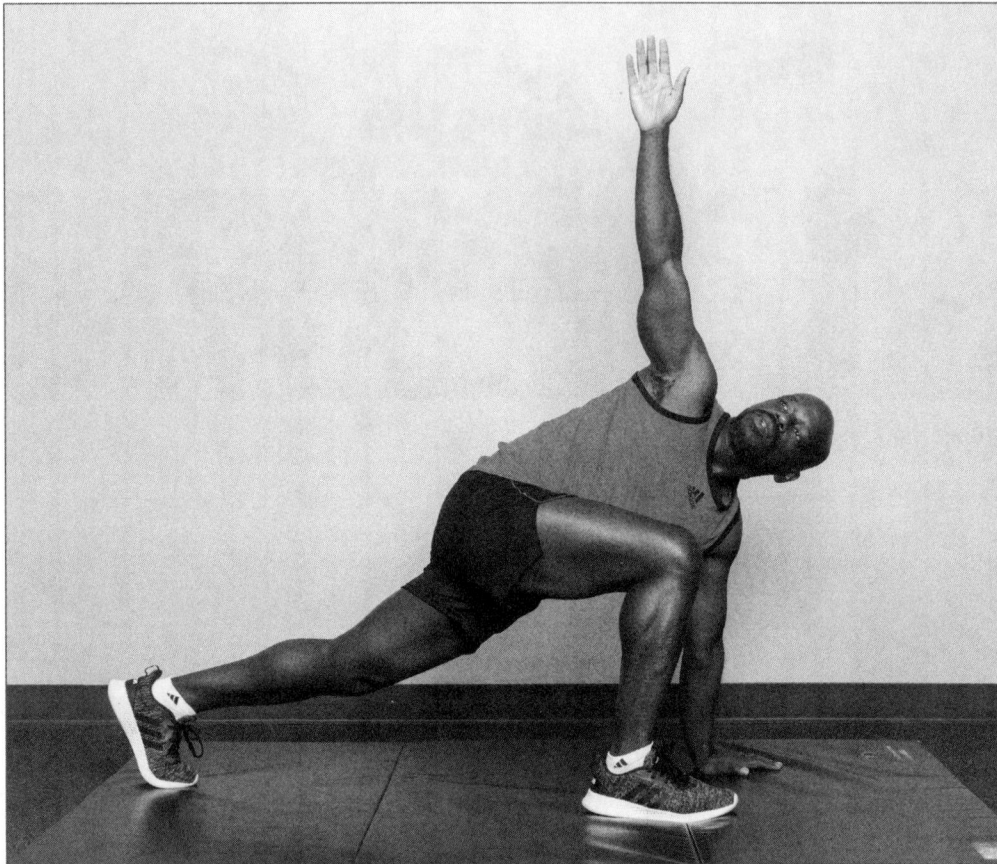

FIGURE 5.6   Hip warm-up: world's greatest stretch.

LIGHTER SETS AS WARM-UP

The limited time you have to train should be spent training, not doing excessive warm-ups. And as the study cited earlier suggested, you want your warm-ups to be specific to the work you are doing. Therefore, I prefer the bulk of my warm-ups to be a light set (or sets) of the exercise that follows. Nothing is a more specific warm-up than that! Often the first set of an exercise or the first several reps of longer sets are also a built-in warm-up, so multiple warm-up sets are likely unnecessary.

When I start training a new client, the first few workouts are *very* light—light enough that the client should be able to perform three sets of 12 to 15 reps on all strength-training exercises without much trouble. These initial workouts aren't designed to be much more challenging than warm-up sets, so I don't find it necessary to go beyond a general warm-up to prepare for these sessions. I start clients so lightly because I want them to practice the proper technique without worrying about finishing the set.

Also, often I won't know until a day or two after a workout if an exercise made someone sore or triggered an adverse reaction. I'd much rather discover this with a lighter weight that has less potential to cause damage.

Only about the last 5 reps of any set (when performed to near failure) provide the stimulus for the body to change and get stronger, meaning that on sets of 12 to 15, the first 7 to 10 reps are basically a warm-up for the later so-called money reps. Why not just do 5 rep sets then? You certainly could. In fact, a classic strength-training protocol is to do 5 sets of 5 reps, called 5 × 5. I sometimes do similar rep schemes with powerlifting clients whose goal is maximum strength. But I think most people, particularly older trainees, should use a higher number of reps with lighter weights to minimize the chance of injury.

As you get stronger, you likely want to do a warm-up set or two on the larger multi-joint exercises like those for chest, back, and thighs, which I place early in the workout. I do not usually find it necessary to warm up for smaller muscle group exercises such as biceps and triceps placed later in the workout, because those muscles have been warmed up from the previous exercises. For example, triceps get warmed up doing pressing exercises for the chest and shoulders, and biceps get warmed up from pulling exercises like chins and rows.

But as I said, there is no one-size-fits-all rule. If your body feels stiff and cold, do a longer warm-up. And if you're going to lift heavy for lower reps, take as many warm-up sets as you need. Because I bench press so heavy most of the time, I need several warm-up sets to prepare for the heavier low-rep sets to come. Unlike high-rep sets, all the heavy reps are money reps, thus there are no built-in warm-up reps early in my work sets. It's up to me to do several progressively heavier warm-up sets to prepare my muscles and joints to lift the heavy work sets and avoid injury.

My warm-up looks like this: 45 pounds × 15 reps, 95 pounds × 10 reps, 135 pounds × 5 reps, 175 pounds × 4 reps, 205 pounds × 3 reps, 225 pounds × 1 to 3 reps. If I'm going heavier than 250 pounds for my work sets, I will continue adding warm-up sets of 1 to 3 reps in 20-pound increments as needed.

That's at least six warm-up sets—whew! But I only do this because of the heavy, low-rep nature of my powerlifting work on the bench press. I will do something similar on competition deadlift, although the weight jumps between warm-up sets will be slightly larger.

Most other big exercises will need one or maybe two warm-up sets at most. For example, on a machine seated row I might do a warm-up set of 90 pounds × 15 reps then jump right to 180-pound work sets. Or I may feel like I need a medium warm-up set of 10 reps at 140 pounds if I'm feeling tight. I rarely do warm-up sets for exercises such as biceps curls or triceps pushdowns unless I'm doing an arm day and thus didn't do any prior chest or back exercises.

WRAPPING UP

I recommend a general warm-up of three to five minutes, ideally on something that moves both your arms and legs, such as an elliptical or fan bike. Picture it like letting that old turntable get up to speed before dropping the needle on the first track—the music sounds cleaner when the gears are already humming. If cranky shoulders or hips are your reality, spin through the mobility drills earlier in this chapter to smooth out the pops and static.

When it's time to lift, remember this rule of thumb: lighter, higher-rep sets are the easy-listening tracks and rarely need their own intro, but heavier, low-rep sets are your arena-rock power chords. Give them an extra riff or two of warm-up. When in doubt, add a little more prep, but remember, a warm-up shouldn't eat up the whole session. Spend only as much time as YOU need so your work sets are ready to rock.

CHAPTER 6

Chest and Back

Remember on Saturday mornings when Prince Adam and Princess Adora raised their Power Swords, called out to Grayskull, and in a crackle of 1980s animation their chests surged, lats flared, and their capes billowed across Eternia? That He-Man/She-Ra transformation is exactly the superhero silhouette we're chasing here: a balanced, mighty chest up front and wing-like lats behind. Only we don't need cartoon lightning to transform our 50-plus bodies, because we have strength training.

"How much can you bench?" was and is still the first question I'm asked, even by non-gymgoers, when the topic of lifting weights comes up. And although the bench press is my favorite exercise and I still enter competitions at age 56 and can bench 300 pounds, that doesn't mean I think the barbell bench press is right for YOU. And if I'm honest, nobody cares how much I can bench press—not even my wife! So if you get asked "how much can you bench?" just remember nobody *really* cares how much you can bench or if you even bench at all. Besides, there are a few good reasons why lifters over 50 may want to avoid the bench press anyway.

For example, one study found that over 66 percent of people aged 51 to 65 had an existing superior labral anterior-posterior (SLAP) tear of the shoulder on an MRI (Lansdown et al. 2018). SLAP tears are a common source of shoulder pain and discomfort, as are other injuries like rotator cuff tears. Very often a SLAP tear will be asymptomatic, and you may not feel any pain . . . until you do the barbell bench press.

Fortunately, there are many exercise options for building the chest other than the barbell bench press and just as many for developing the back so we shouldn't be deterred from our Masters of the Universe-like transformation regardless of our ability to perform a particular exercise. From barbells and dumbbells to machine, cable, and body-weight exercise variations, this chapter includes numerous options to ensure both a comprehensive workout and appropriate alternatives should a certain exercise be contraindicated for you. As always, proper form and technique are essential for maximizing muscle growth and minimizing the risk of injury, so pay close attention to the descriptions provided.

CHEST EXERCISES

A strong, muscular chest has always been a hallmark of good strength and fitness. Unfortunately, underdeveloped pecs can be a problem area for those of us over 50, where time and gravity have shifted everything lower. Strength training (and low body-fat levels) can help prevent the dreaded "man boobs" every guy fears and can also provide a good muscular "antigravity" foundation for women's chests.

There are two general types of chest exercises: pressing motions and flying motions. Pressing motions like push-ups and bench-press variations also heavily involve muscles of the shoulder and triceps and thus will allow for the use of heavier weights. Flying motions attempt to minimize the help of those other muscles and focus directly on the pecs. Pressing variations can carry greater risk because of the loads used, but flying motions should also be used with caution because too great a range of motion in the stretch position can lead to shoulder pain. Just because you're over 50 doesn't mean you can't do an exercise (as mentioned, I still bench press 300 pounds at age 56), but it does mean you should be cautious and refrain from using exercises or loads that cause you joint pain.

Dumbbell Bench Press

The dumbbell bench press is likely a better option for the trainee over 50 than the barbell version. It's a versatile exercise in that you can find the ideal elbow and wrist position that works for you while pressing, while the barbell keeps you in a more fixed position that may not be right for you. Because of the flexibility of arm positions (and the fact that there is no barbell to stop you at the chest), dumbbells can allow for a greater range of motion without causing the shoulder irritation the barbell can. Another benefit is that because you have a separate weight in each hand, your stability will be challenged more than with the barbell. This is great for the stabilizer muscles of the shoulder but will naturally cause you to use lighter weights than you would use with the barbell bench press. For example, I can bench press 300 pounds on a barbell bench press, but I can't budge 150-pound dumbbells.

INSTRUCTION

- Lie down on a flat bench (or a very slight incline [10-15 degrees] if you have an adjustable bench) with a dumbbell in each hand. Walk the shoulder blades together and elevate the chest.
- Position the dumbbells at chest level, with your palms facing in (figure *a*).
- Press the dumbbells up until your arms are fully extended (figure *b*). You may keep the dumbbells facing each other or rotate them inward (palms down toward the feet) as you press. The neutral, palms-in grip is usually better for those who feel shoulder pain while pressing. As with the barbell bench press, think "stacked wrists, elbows, and shoulders" at extension.
- Slowly lower the dumbbells back to the starting position.
- Repeat for the desired number of repetitions.

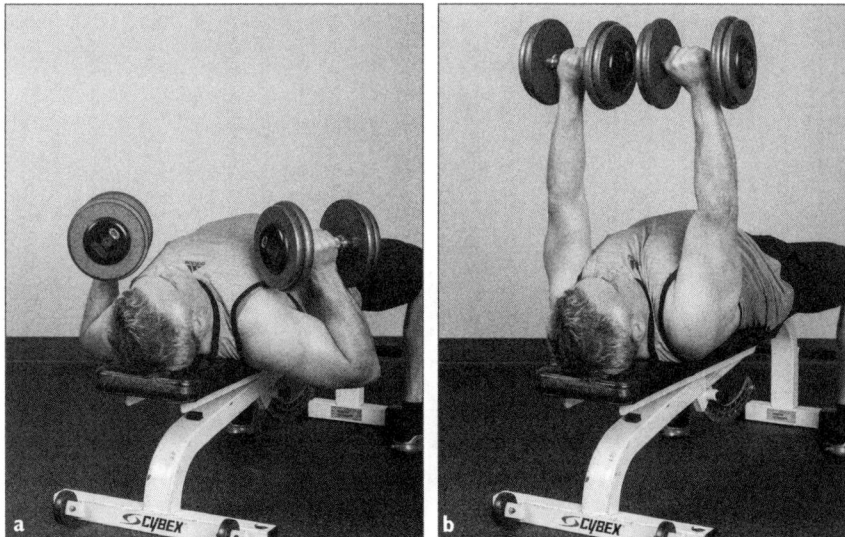

CHAD'S TAKE

I prefer to do the dumbbell chest press at a very slight incline (about 10 degrees), rather than completely flat. Do not confuse this with the steeper angles (30 to 45 degrees) of the incline dumbbell press. I do this because it tends to feel more comfortable than completely flat and because it's a bit easier to sit up with heavy dumbbells at the end of my set. I've found dumbbells to be a better option than a barbell for most people over 50 because the dumbbells allow you to find the right elbow and wrist position for your specific aches and pains or range of motion limitations.

Barbell Bench Press

The barbell bench press is a staple exercise for building chest strength and mass. It targets the pectoral muscles, as well as engaging the triceps and anterior deltoids as secondary muscles. It is *highly* recommended that you use a spotter when barbell bench pressing. At a minimum, bench at a power rack or with safety stands that will prevent you from getting crushed should something go wrong.

INSTRUCTION

- Lie down on a flat bench with your feet flat on the floor. Your eyes should be directly under the barbell.
- "Walk" your shoulder blades together (imagine pulling them back and down) and push the chest up. This helps to set your shoulder girdle to provide stability for the pressing to come.
- Grasp the barbell with a grip slightly wider than shoulder width (figure *a*). (You can try various width grips to see what feels best for you, but avoid the extremes of too wide or too narrow.)
- Unrack the barbell and lower it slowly to your lower to midchest, keeping elbows in at roughly a 30- to 45-degree angle with the body (figure *b*). (Note: Some people will do better to stop an inch or two above the chest to avoid shoulder strain if they lack the pain-free range of motion to touch the chest. This is OK!)
- Push the barbell back up until your arms are extended but leaving the elbows unlocked, ideally with the wrists, elbows, and shoulders stacked in vertical alignment.
- Repeat for the desired number of repetitions.

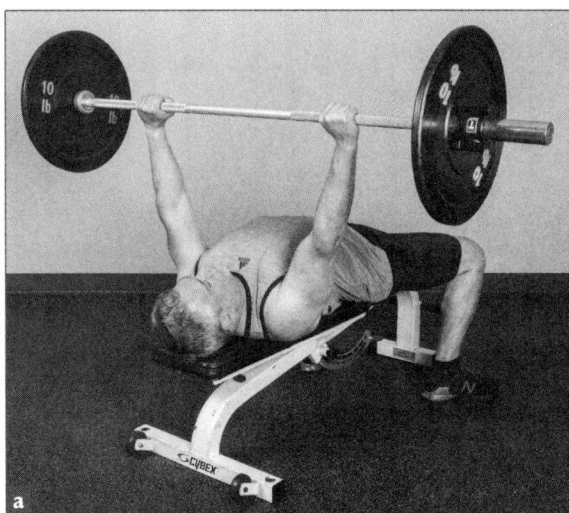

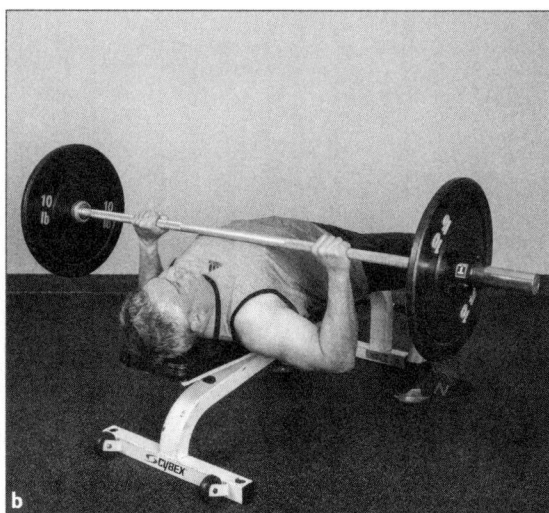

CHAD'S TAKE

The temptation to go too heavy, especially for those over 50 who "benched 225 in high school," is common. There's nothing inherently wrong with the barbell bench press for those of us over 50. Heck, I coached a client, Barbara Radwin-Garmon, to a World Bench Press Championship gold medal in 2013 when she was 70 years old! But as fulfilling as it is to bench press more weight than people half your age (as I've done in many meets), you must use a slow and steady approach to benching heavier.

As with any exercise, don't bench press if it causes pain, especially in the shoulders (an area ripe for injury when barbell bench pressing). Start light and progress slowly, avoiding the urge to pile on more weight too quickly. A great way to ensure you don't go too heavy is to pause your reps for a second at the bottom (on the chest or even slightly above). This will prevent using momentum to aid in performing the lift and will lead to much greater strength in a bench competition, should you ever try masters powerlifting. Similarly, never bounce the bar off your chest—always control the weight; don't let the weight control you. Lastly, if you aren't in a powerlifting competition, you don't have to touch your chest with the barbell if it causes you pain. I've had clients who were OK to bench press if they stopped an inch or two above the chest but felt shoulder pain doing the full range of motion. While we strive to do a full range of motion on every exercise, those of us over 50 should be particularly aware of using the fullest range that we can that also doesn't cause us joint pain.

Machine Chest Press

The chest press machine is a shoulder-friendly alternative to free weights for targeting the chest muscles. These machines require less stability and control than their free-weight counterparts, which not only makes it easier on the shoulders but also allows for more weight while targeting the pecs. I especially like Hammer Strength equipment and have their machines at my gym. They have independent right and left arms, which can help keep the dominant side from doing a bit more work than the nondominant side as can happen with traditional fixed-handle machines. Another bonus of machines is that they are designed to make a spotter unnecessary.

INSTRUCTION

- Adjust the seat height so that the handles are aligned with your midchest.
- Sit with your back firmly against the backrest and grasp the handles with your palms facing forward (figure a). Walk shoulder blades together.
- Press the handles forward until your arms are extended, taking care not to lock out the elbows (figure b).
- Slowly return the handles to the starting position. To keep tension on the muscles being used, do not allow the weight stack to touch between reps.
- Repeat for the desired number of repetitions.

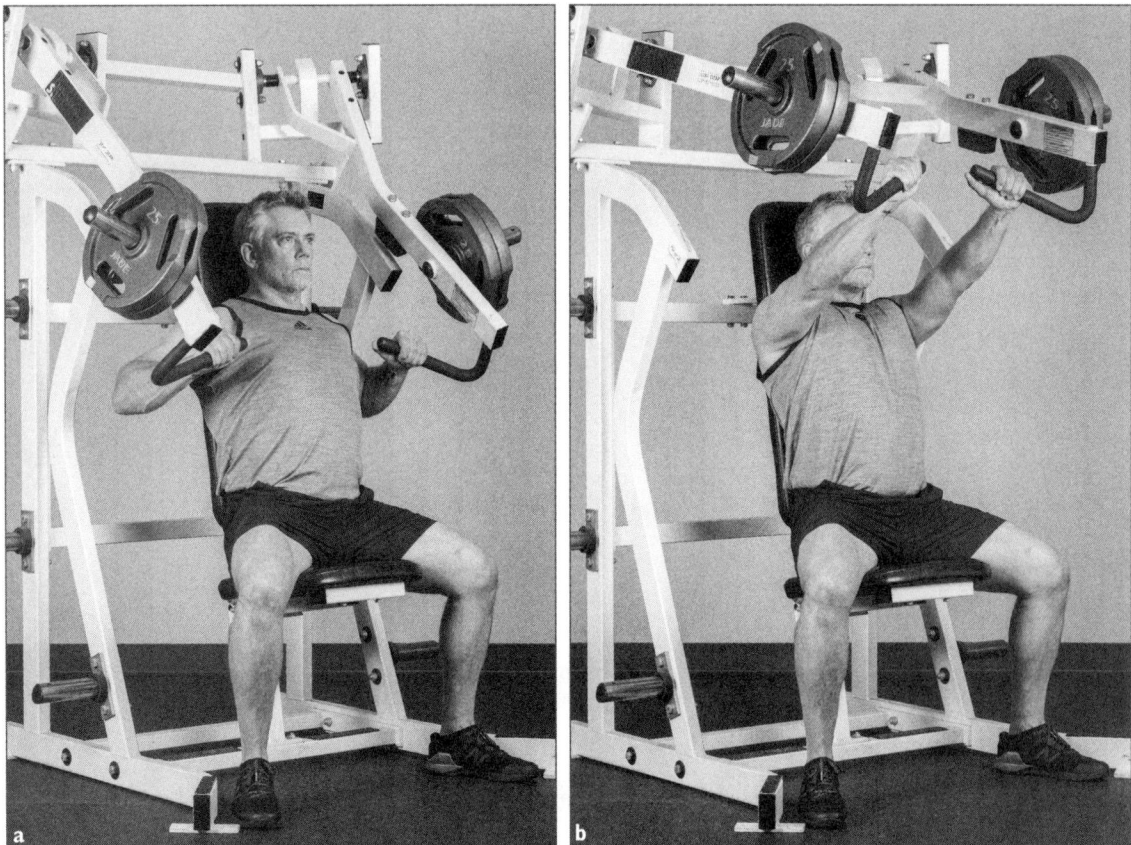

CHAD'S TAKE

An often overlooked benefit of machines is the ability to safely work more explosively than with free weights. This is due to the extra stability the fixed path of the machine provides, allowing you to do the positive portion of the rep explosively, trying to accelerate the weights on the way up. While it's good to perform free-weight exercise with an explosive positive, I find it safer to do on machines, especially if you don't have a spotter.

Why is training explosively important? The ability to express our strength quickly diminishes even quicker than our strength as we age. While strength and power may seem synonymous to the layperson, they are distinct abilities. Strength is how much we can lift; power is a combination of how much we can lift *and* how quickly we can lift it. A lack of power can make it impossible for our muscles to produce force quickly, something needed to stand up from a chair or jump out of the way in an emergency. Studies show that using somewhat lighter weights that can be lifted quickly is one of the few ways we know to mitigate these age-related power losses (Reid and Fielding 2012). It's another reason why I prefer to use sets of at least 8 and usually more like 10 to 15 reps. I can move these weights faster and retain my ability to produce power. I always tell my clients that even if the positive part of the rep isn't moving fast, think "fast" on the way up. Try to move it as quickly as you can in good form.

Push-Up

The push-up is a classic body-weight exercise that targets the chest muscles while also engaging the triceps and shoulders. It's also a great core exercise because it's basically a moving plank. Don't make the mistake of assuming this is a beginner exercise. Push-ups can be very difficult to perform correctly. They are also a great option to improve your power because you can push up as explosively as possible. You may even be able to do plyometric push-ups (like clapping push-ups), providing your joints are OK absorbing the force of the landing.

INSTRUCTION

- Begin in a plank position, hands on the floor (or a bar; see Chad's Take) about shoulder-width or slightly wider apart, balls of the feet on the ground. Slightly tuck the pelvis and brace the core (figure *a*).
- Lower your body by bending your elbows until your chest nearly touches the ground or bar. Keep the elbows between 30 and 45 degrees from the side. They should *not* flare out 90 degrees, a common error that can cause shoulder pain or worse (figure *b*).
- Push yourself back up to the starting position.
- Repeat for the desired number of repetitions.

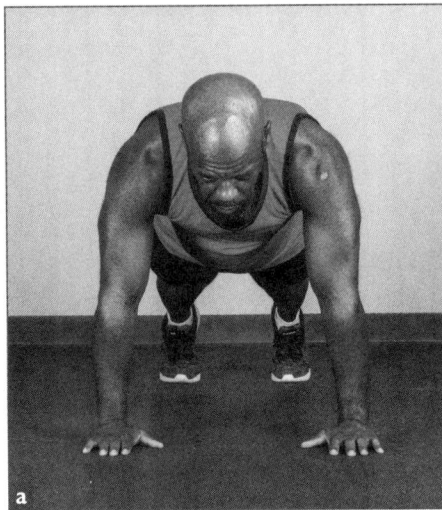

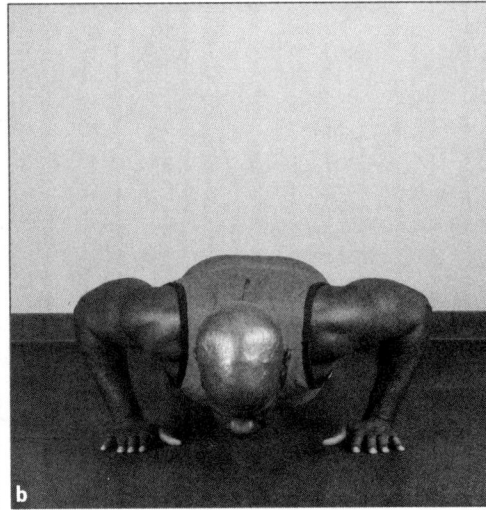

CHAD'S TAKE

In addition to benefiting the pecs, shoulders, and triceps, push-ups are also a great exercise to work the serratus anterior, an important stabilizer of the scapula. The serratus sits on the side of your rib cage and helps to keep your shoulder blade back and down, thus countering the hunched, shoulders-rolled-forward position many people have. But it only works if you fully extend your arms at the top of the push-up. This is called *scapular protraction* or *abduction*. Imagine pulling your shoulder blades apart and around the rib cage, like a cat stretch in yoga, but without the need to arch your back. My cue is to push your rib cage back through your shoulder blades at the top of the movement. Some folks call this a "push-up plus"; I just call it good push-up form.

However, many people will not be able to start doing this style of push-up from the ground, so I use an adjustable power rack and often start clients at whatever height and angle I need to allow them to perform the push-up in this way. The rack allows the client to lift less of their body weight while learning proper form. I then slowly lower the bar on the power rack until the clients can do push-ups properly from the floor. Note: Even if you can do push-ups from the floor, you may not have the wrist flexibility to do so comfortably. Use push-up handles or even hexagonal dumbbells (they won't roll) to allow the wrist to stay more neutral. Place them at a width and angle comfortable on your wrists and shoulders that allows you to continue using the proper form. For most people the hands will be directly under the shoulders at the top of the push-up.

Cable Crossover

The cable crossover is a versatile exercise that targets the chest muscles with constant tension throughout the movement. There are many great variations based on pulley height and angle of pull. Traditionally, bodybuilders have done the crossover with the pulleys set high and drawing the cables down to meet in front of the body near the waist as shown here. However, you can set the cables low and pull up and across your face. You could set the cables at chest level and mimic a similar form to the pec deck. Feel free to play around with the pulley height and the angle of pull and see what feels best on your shoulders while allowing you to connect to the pec muscles.

INSTRUCTION

- Adjust the pulleys to your desired height and attach handles to both sides.
- Grasp the handles with your palms facing forward and step forward to create tension in the cables (figure a). If you have a traditional cable crossover machine, you will be in between each weight stack. If you use a functional trainer machine that has two arms coming out of one central base, you'll be facing away from the machine.
- With a slight bend in your elbows, bring your hands together in front of your chest. There is no need to cross the handles; simply try to touch the handles together (figure b).
- Slowly return your hands to the starting position, maintaining tension in the cables.
- Repeat for the desired number of repetitions.

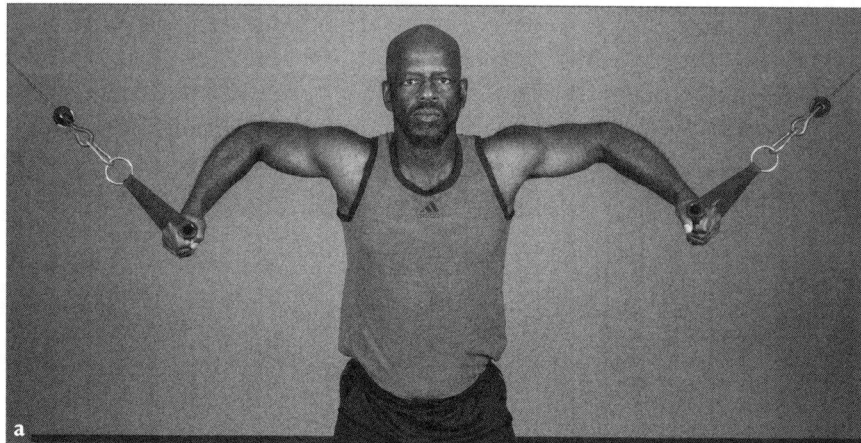

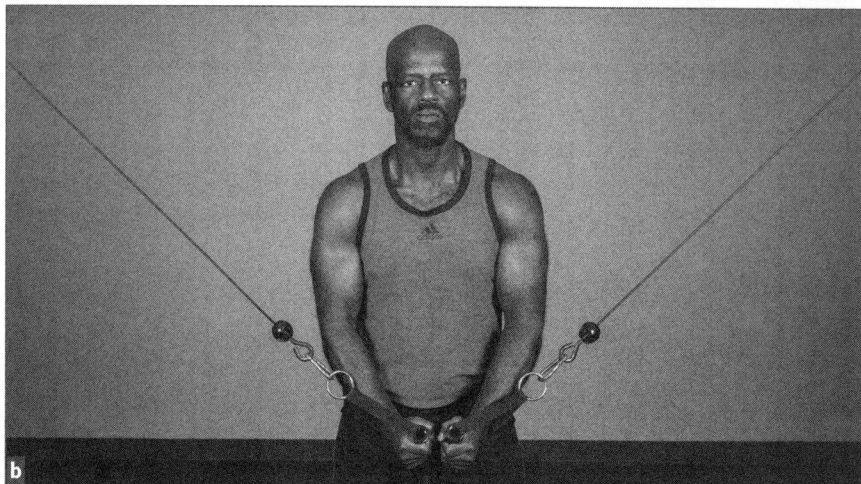

CHAD'S TAKE

I *love* cables for chest growth. They are a great substitute for dumbbell flying motions because the cables allow for continuous tension on the pecs throughout the range of motion, which is not possible with free weights. You can do them standing or seated, if you prefer. As mentioned before, you can also set the pulleys high and pull low in front, or you can set them low and pull high. I especially like the low pulley to head height crossover because it accentuates the upper pecs near the collarbone more. I find the other variations to be a bit redundant since I do a ton of bench pressing. Play around and find what you like best!

Pec Deck Fly

The pec deck fly is an isolation exercise that targets the pectoral muscles. As I mentioned in the beginning of this section, flying motions, while great for targeting the pecs, can put the shoulder joint in a precarious position, so I prefer to do machine flies because they can be safer and easier to control than dumbbells. Most pec decks have a range-of-motion limiter you can set to prevent overstretching the shoulder joint. I find this especially beneficial for those of us over 50 because of those previously mentioned SLAP tears.

INSTRUCTION

- Adjust the seat height of the machine for optimal comfort and positioning. Depending on the style of pec deck (handles versus forearm pads) you'll want to set the seat at a height that puts the handles (or your elbow if using vertical forearm pads) at the same level as the shoulder or slightly lower. Use what feels best on your shoulders. Set the range limiter (if available) at a point where the upper arm stops in line with the chest and shoulders.
- Sit with your back firmly against the backrest and grasp the handles with your palms facing inward (figure a). (Or place your forearms hands up against the vertical pads.)
- Bring the handles together in front of your chest, squeezing your pectoral muscles at the end of the movement (figure b).
- Slowly return the handles to the starting position.
- Repeat for the desired number of repetitions.

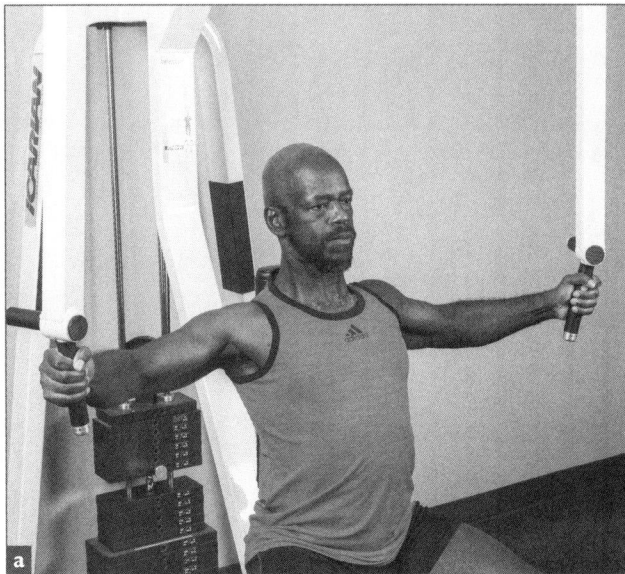 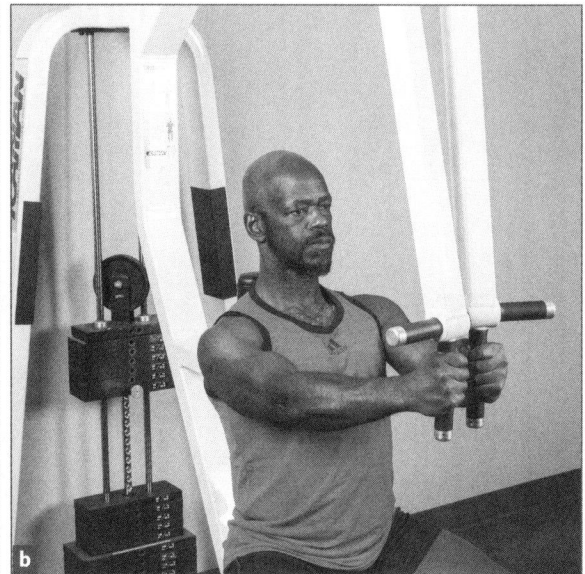

CHAD'S TAKE

I keep my butt a bit out from the back pad and arch my back to elevate my chest. I feel a better connection to the pecs in this position. Also, on machines that have pivoting handles, I keep my elbows bent in the stretched position but then straighten and reach in the contracted position to further engage the pecs. As a lifter over 50 whose shoulders can get cranky from all the heavy benching I do, I find the pec deck fly to be the perfect option to target my pecs while taking it easy on my shoulders and requiring no triceps help, something that can be limiting on pressing motions.

Incline Dumbbell Bench Press

As with the incline barbell bench press, this exercise targets the upper chest muscles while allowing for a greater range of motion than the incline barbell. As with the flat dumbbell bench press, you'll likely need to use much lighter weights than with the barbell counterpart because of the instability resulting from having a dumbbell in each hand. And again, be cautious of overstretching the shoulder joint at the bottom of the movement—dumbbells allow for a greater range of motion than barbells.

INSTRUCTION

- Set up an incline bench at a 30- to 45-degree angle. Walk the shoulder blades together and elevate the chest.
- Position the dumbbells at chest level, with your palms facing in (figure a).
- Press the dumbbells up until your arms are fully extended (figure b). You may keep the dumbbells facing each other or rotate them inward (palms down toward the feet) as you press. The neutral, palms-in grip is usually better for those who feel shoulder pain while pressing. As with the barbell bench press, think "stacked wrists, elbows, and shoulders" at extension.
- Slowly lower the dumbbells back to the starting position.
- Repeat for the desired number of repetitions.

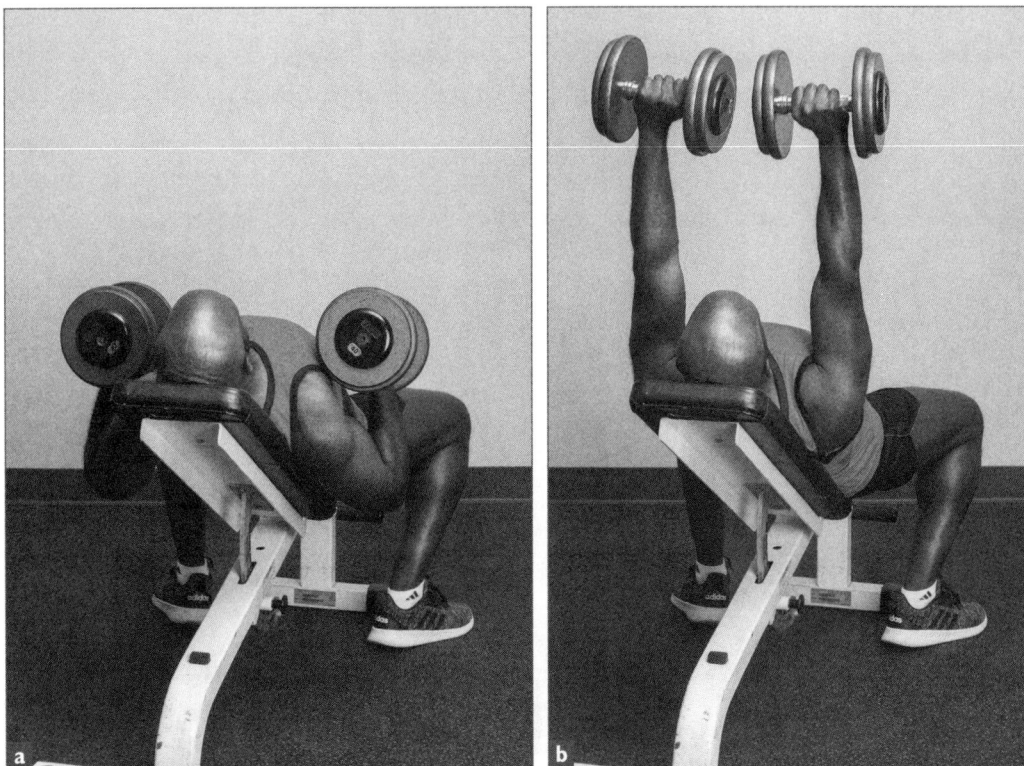

CHAD'S TAKE

I tend to keep my palms at an angle to my body throughout the range of motion—neither completely neutral nor palms down, nor with any rotation of the dumbbells. I find this allows me to have better stability and focus during the exercise. For those over 50 with existing shoulder pain, the parallel, palms-facing-in grip will likely cause the least shoulder irritation and minimize the risk of further injury.

Incline Barbell Bench Press

The incline barbell bench press targets the upper chest muscles, with some emphasis on the anterior deltoids and triceps. The incline barbell bench press is like the flat barbell bench press with nearly identical cues and safety concerns, especially the preference to use a spotter. I find it a bit redundant to include a flat bench press version and an incline bench press variation in the same workout (something seen heavily in bodybuilding magazines in the '80s and '90s). Just pick one or the other and focus on doing it well.

INSTRUCTION

- Set up an incline bench at a 30- to 45-degree angle. It's OK to try different angles and see what you like best. You may even prefer to train from multiple angles.

- Walk your shoulder blades together (think pulling them back and down) and push the chest up. This helps to set your shoulder girdle and provide stability for the pressing to come.

- Grasp the barbell with a grip slightly wider than shoulder width. (You can try various width grips to see what feels best for you, but avoid the extremes of too wide or too narrow.)

- Unrack the barbell (figure *a*) and lower it slowly to your lower to midchest, keeping your elbows in at roughly a 30- to 45-degree angle with the body (figure *b*). (Note: Some people will do better to stop an inch or two above the chest to avoid shoulder strain if they lack the pain-free range of motion to touch the chest. This is OK!)

- Push the barbell back up until your arms are extended but leaving the elbows unlocked, ideally with the wrists, elbows, and shoulders stacked in vertical alignment.

- Repeat for the desired number of repetitions.

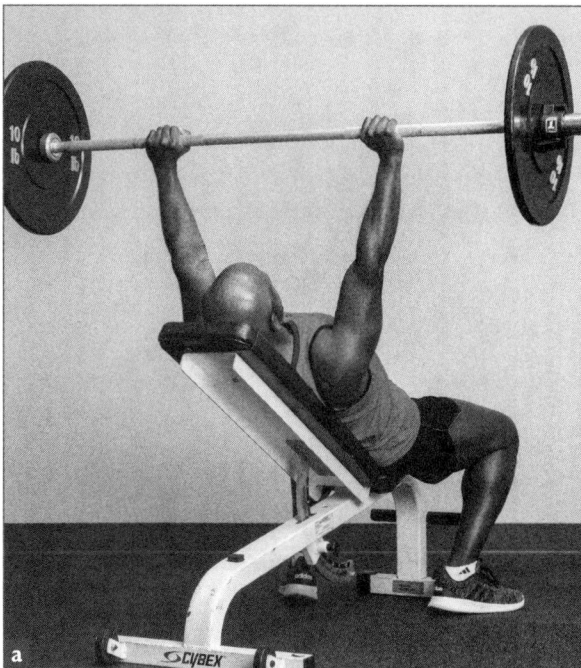 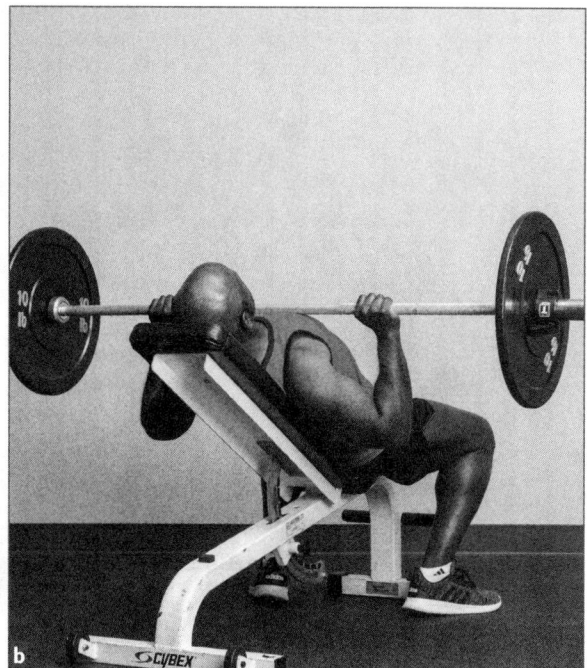

CHAD'S TAKE

If you have access to a Smith machine, use it with the incline barbell bench press. With similar bar paths, the Smith machine can provide the benefits of the incline barbell bench press with less concern about balance and stability and allowing for more focus on the pecs. This can be a great option for us over-50 trainees who have existing shoulder issues. Note: I do not like the Smith machine in place of the flat barbell bench press because the bar paths are too dissimilar, in my opinion.

Incline Dumbbell Fly

This isolation exercise targets the upper chest muscles and engages the pectoral muscles through a different movement pattern than a press. I prefer to do incline flys with the cable crossover machine and an adjustable bench rather than with dumbbells because of the continuous tension provided by the cables.

INSTRUCTION

- Set up an incline bench at a 30- to 45-degree angle.
- Lie down on the bench with a dumbbell in each hand.
- Start with the dumbbells directly above your chest, with your palms facing each other and a slight bend in your elbows (figure *a*).
- Slowly lower the dumbbells out to your sides, maintaining the slight bend in your elbows and feeling a stretch in your chest muscles (figure *b*).
- Bring the dumbbells back to the starting position, squeezing your chest muscles at the top of the movement.
- Repeat for the desired number of repetitions.

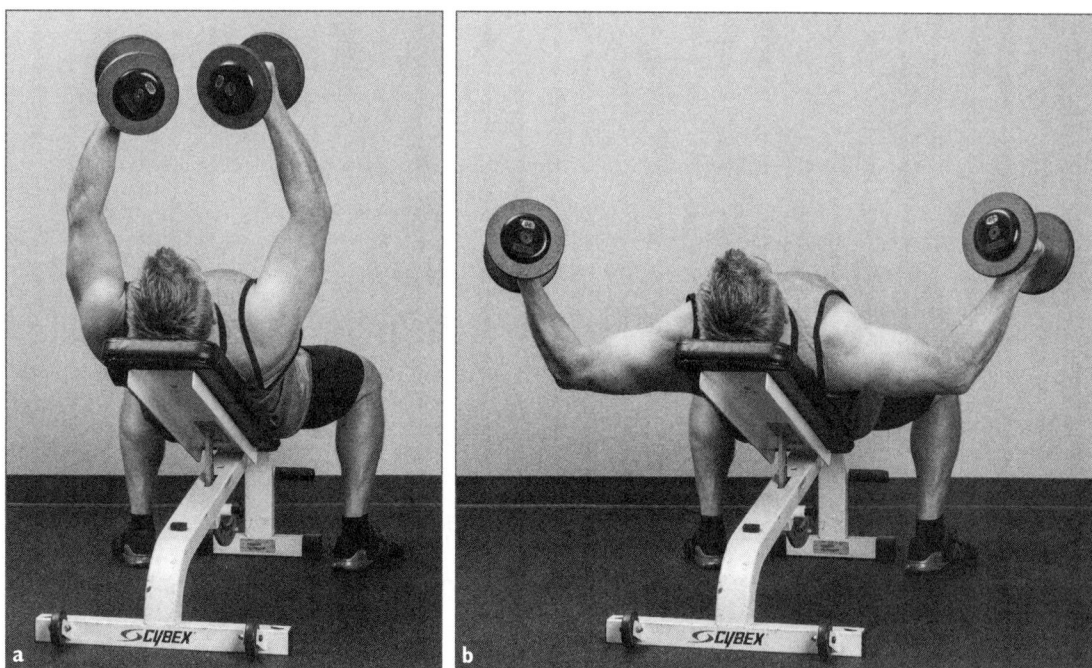

CHAD'S TAKE

One great way to perform incline dumbbell flys is to use a flying motion on the way down (the negative), then pull the dumbbells into the sides of the chest and do an incline dumbbell press on the way up (the positive). This option will allow you to use heavier weights than a strict fly, so pay careful attention to lowering the dumbbells under control and not overstretching at the bottom.

Incline dumbbell flys can also be great to pair with incline dumbbell presses as a pre-exhaust superset (isolation movement followed immediately by a compound movement for the same muscles). This allows you to get more out of a lighter weight because you've "pre-exhausted" the larger chest muscles with the flys. These are great techniques for the athlete over 50 whose shoulder issues limit the amount of weight they can use safely.

Cable Squeeze Press

This chest isolation exercise targets the pecs in a unique way because you press the cable handles together as you press the weight up. This promotes a really intense muscle contraction, and I find it a great option for those who have a hard time "connecting" to the pecs during traditional pressing motions. There are aspects of both the sagittal and transverse plane working on the squeeze press that I really like. They can also be performed using dumbbells on either a flat or incline bench, or you can do them standing when using cables, which you cannot do when using dumbbells.

INSTRUCTION

- Adjust the pulleys to chest level and attach handles to both sides.
- Grasp the handles with your palms facing forward and step forward to create tension in the cables. If you have a traditional cable crossover machine you will be in between each weight stack. If you use a functional trainer machine that has two arms coming out of one central base, you'll be facing away from the machine. Bring the handles together directly in front of the chest (touching) with the arms against your sides (figure *a*).
- Press your hands forward and together to extend fully in front of your chest. Make sure the handles stay in contact. You should aim to squeeze the handles together while you press (figure *b*).
- Slowly return your hands to the starting position, maintaining tension in the cables and again ensuring the handles stay touching throughout.
- Repeat for the desired number of repetitions.

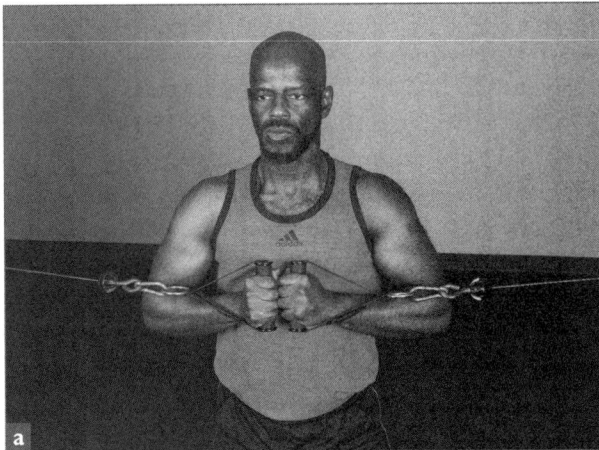

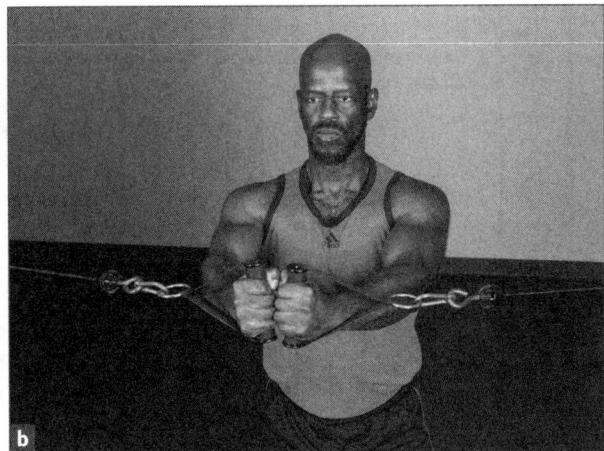

CHAD'S TAKE
I really like the squeeze press for the over-50 crowd because the arm position is very friendly to older shoulders, and it's another technique that allows for good results using lighter weights. I like to do these seated with the bench anywhere from nearly vertical with pulleys at chest height (will be like lying flat with pulleys at lowest setting), and anywhere down to about a 30-degree angle, lowering the pulleys as the angle of the bench goes down. Another fun way to do these is to squeeze press on the positive portion of the rep and cable fly during the negative portion, similar to the dumbbell fly variation mentioned previously.

BACK EXERCISES

A well-developed back is a rare sight to behold. Unfortunately, many trainees pay less attention to the muscles of the back simply because they don't see them in the mirror, but they are doing themselves a disservice. There are many muscles on the back sides of our bodies—lats, traps, rhomboids, spinal erectors, teres major, rear delts—and they all should be strong and well developed.

From an aesthetic standpoint (and who doesn't want to look their best over age 50?), a well-built back signals a youthfulness and vitality that defies our years. Men are generally most concerned with the V-taper, the wide-shouldered, narrow-waisted look of your average superhero. But female trainees, while not typically looking for the same dimensions as male trainees, still benefit from a strong, defined back.

I remember going to the wedding of a female client two decades ago in New Orleans. As she walked down the aisle in her backless wedding dress, the revelation of her toned, defined back muscles elicited an audible gasp from the crowd! It was one of the proudest moments of my career.

Back exercises generally fall into two main categories: rowing motions and pull-down or pull-up motions. Rowing is a "horizontal pull," and pull-downs and pull-ups are a "vertical pull." Body-weight back exercises like pull-ups or inverted rows are extremely difficult, so ideally, you'll have access to machines or cables for both types of pulls, or even barbells or dumbbells for certain rowing exercises.

One aspect of back training you may have encountered is whether or not to use wrist straps to enhance your grip on pulling exercises. I try not to use them because I want my forearms and grip strength to be as strong as my back. But some people may find that on their heaviest sets their grip strength gives out long before their back muscles are fatigued. In that instance, I'd recommend not using straps on most sets. You definitely shouldn't need them on warm-up sets, and probably not on the first set or two of your work sets. So use them sparingly, only as needed, to ensure your grip doesn't get weaker from reliance on straps.

Pendlay Row

The Pendlay row is an excellent compound exercise for targeting the upper and middle back muscles. However, if you have a chest-supported row (machine, T-bar row, or seal row bench), this would be the preferred option because it better supports the core.

INSTRUCTION

- Stand with your feet shoulder-width apart, knees slightly bent.
- Grasp the barbell with an overhand grip, hands slightly wider than shoulder width. (Note: You can use an underhand grip if it is more comfortable for you.)
- Bend forward at the hips until your torso is roughly parallel to the floor (figure *a*).
- Pull the barbell toward your lower chest, keeping your elbows close to your body, aiming to touch the chest on each repetition (figure *b*).
- Slowly lower the barbell back down to the starting position.
- Repeat for the desired number of repetitions.

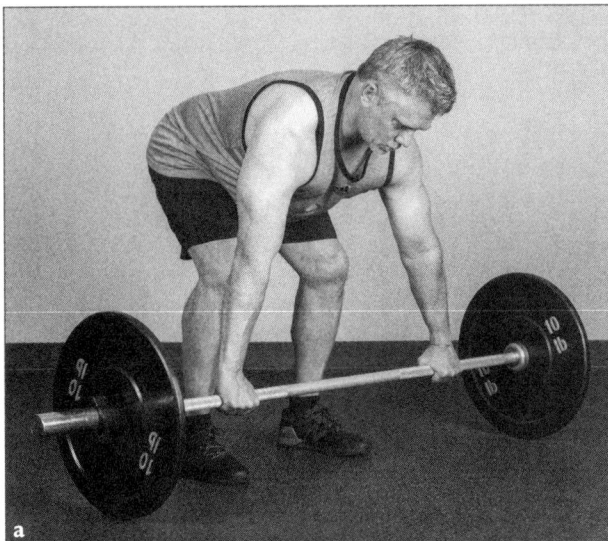

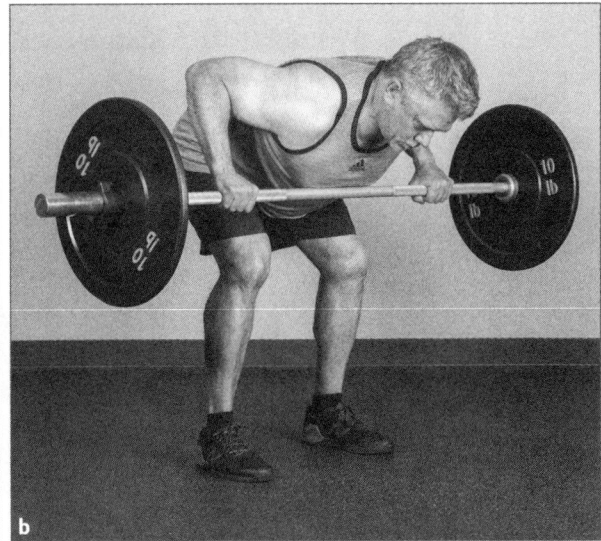

CHAD'S TAKE

I prefer the Pendlay row (named after famed Olympic weightlifting coach Glenn Pendlay) over traditional bent-over barbell rows. The Pendlay row uses a slightly wider grip than a traditional row. You also finish each rep on the floor and quickly reset between reps. I find this reset a particular advantage of the Pendlay row, in that it allows you to really focus on engaging your upper back muscles, while potentially taking stress off the low back by not having the weight suspended the entire set. I also like to do a slight pause at the chest. This forces me to use lighter weights and actually control the movement with my upper back muscles more fully.

Machine Seated Row

The machine seated row is an effective exercise for targeting the middle and upper back muscles and is another great choice of chest-supported row. It is my single favorite back exercise. I especially like machines where the left and right handle are independent of each other like the Hammer Strength Iso-Lateral line of equipment I have at my studio. This keeps the dominant side from being able to do more work than the weak side.

INSTRUCTION

- Adjust the seat height and chest pad for optimal comfort and positioning.
- Sit with your chest against the chest pad and grasp the handles with an overhand grip (figure *a*).
- Pull the handles toward your lower chest, squeezing your shoulder blades together at the end of the movement (figure *b*). Note: Once the upper arm is aligned with the body, finish the squeeze by elevating the chest and pulling the shoulder blades together, paying careful attention not to pull the elbows back behind the body too far so that the shoulder tips forward, which can lead to shoulder pain and injury.
- Slowly return the handles to the starting position.
- Repeat for the desired number of repetitions.

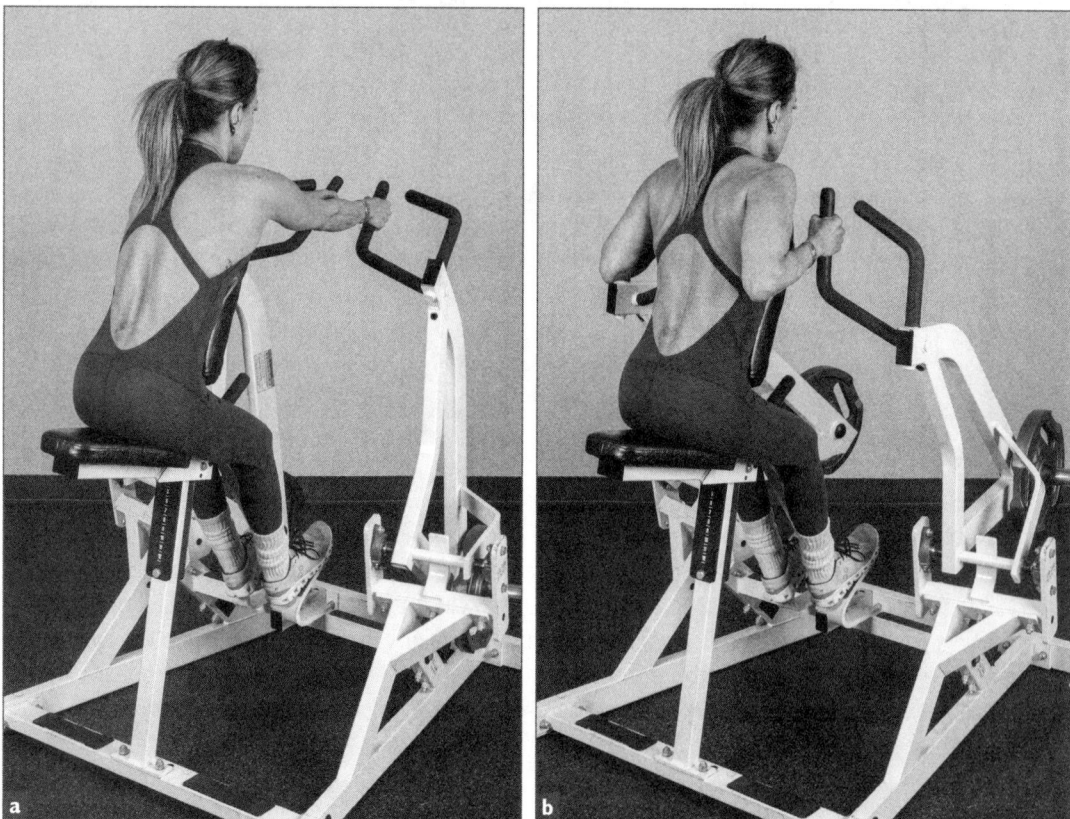

CHAD'S TAKE

I use two cues with clients that I believe are critical to get the most out of this exercise:

1. When initiating the row, draw the shoulders back as far as possible without bending the elbows (think shrugging backward). I really want you to connect to the back muscles and not just the biceps. When you've drawn the shoulders back as far as you can, bend the elbows and continue to pull the weights back until you've brought the shoulder blades together.

2. Always keep the chest against the pad. Do not get tempted to lean back and put momentum into the lift. It's easy to turn this great exercise into a crummy biceps exercise or a lower back thrasher.

Two-Dumbbell Chest-Supported Row

This exercise is a dumbbell variation of the bent-over barbell row that targets the same muscle groups. Again, an advantage to dumbbells is not having a fixed grip on a single barbell; therefore, you can pull with a wrist angle that's most comfortable for you. Also, you may be able to get slightly more range of motion at the top position since you won't have a barbell hitting your torso.

INSTRUCTION

- Stand with your feet shoulder-width apart, knees slightly bent.
- Hold a dumbbell in each hand with a neutral to overhand grip.
- Lie face down on an incline bench with your chest supported by the bench and your head off the end (figure a).
- Pull the dumbbells toward your lower chest, keeping your elbows close to your body (figure b).
- Slowly lower the dumbbells back down to the starting position.
- Repeat for the desired number of repetitions.

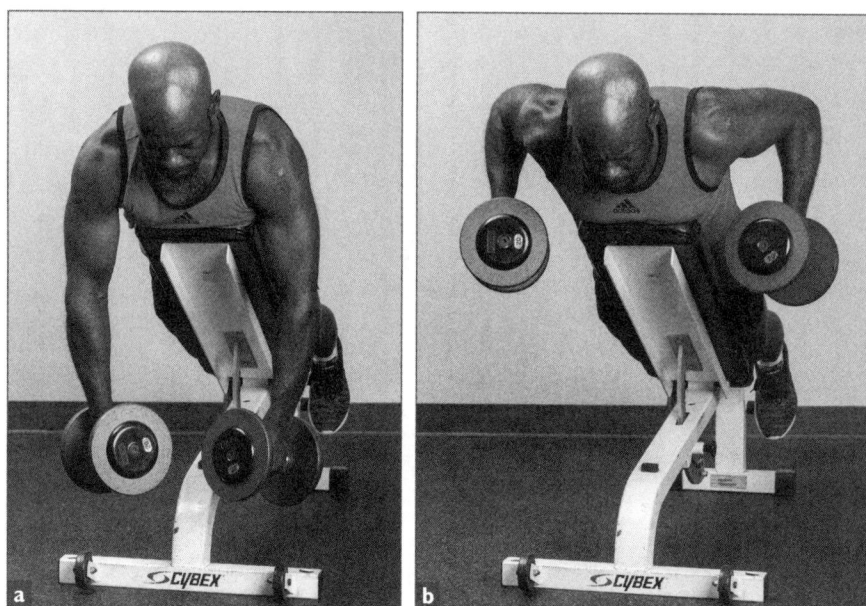

CHAD'S TAKE

While you could do these Pendlay style off the floor, I much prefer doing them face down on an incline bench at a 30- to 45-degree angle. I will always choose a chest-supported row over an unsupported one if available. Again, a slight pause in the top contracted position is a great option. I also like to use a more arcing motion with my arms (think mirror image of a dumbbell fly) rather than pulling straight up. I keep a neutral or slightly pronated grip and keep the elbows at about a 30- to 45-degree angle from my sides—basically a mirror image of my bench press using the opposing muscles. I find this allows me to better target the upper back muscles while minimizing reliance on the smaller biceps muscles.

Lat Pull-Down

The lat pull-down is a compound exercise that targets the latissimus dorsi and other muscles in the upper back. Cable machines have various attachments that employ an array of grip widths and angles. The form is basically the same for all variations, so feel free to use the attachments that are most comfortable for you and try other options occasionally. Note that there is no training benefit to using an extremely wide grip—a wide grip does not equal a wide back, but it could prove injurious to your shoulder joint over time.

INSTRUCTION

- Adjust the seat height and leg pads for optimal comfort and positioning. The thigh pads should be snug against the top of your leg to keep you anchored when using heavier weights. On some machines the adjustment is done via the thigh pads, and on others the thigh pad is fixed and the seat adjusts, while some machines don't have thigh pads at all.
- If using a traditional straight lat pull-down bar, grasp the bar with a shoulder-width, overhand grip. If using a neutral-grip bar, grasp it with your palms facing inward (figure a).
- Pull the bar down to your upper chest, squeezing your shoulder blades together at the end of the movement (figure b).
- Slowly return the bar to the starting position.
- Repeat for the desired number of repetitions.

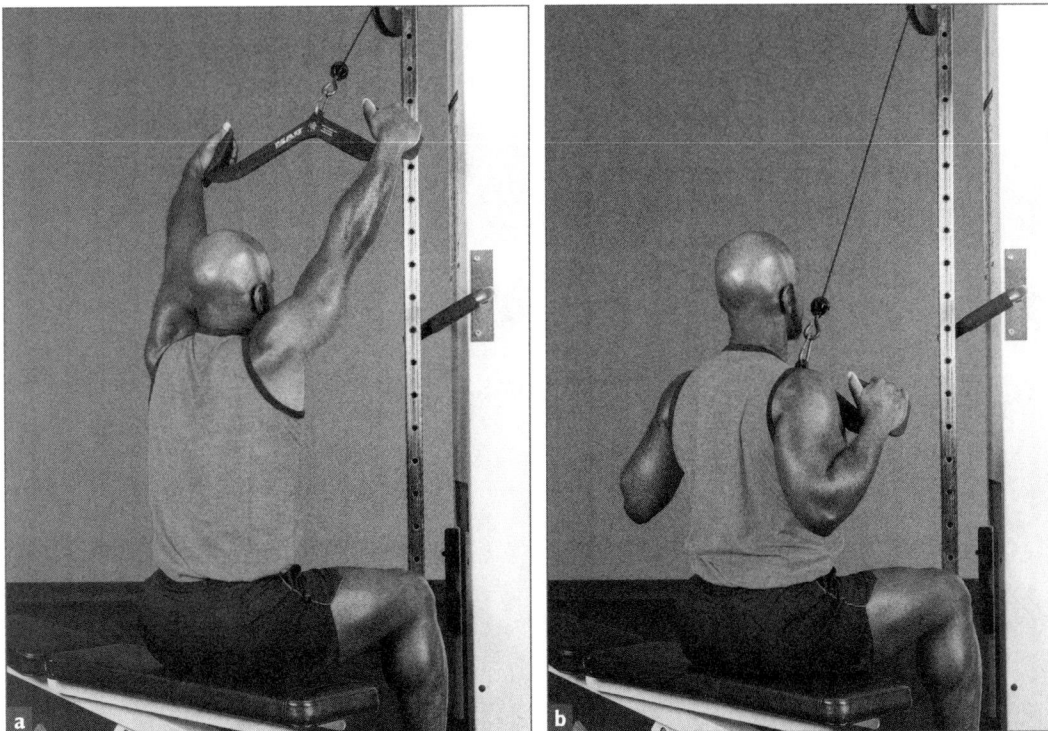

CHAD'S TAKE

The lat pull-down is your best bet if you haven't done a body-weight pull-up since Ronald Reagan was president. I love the variety with this exercise and use a half dozen different attachments at my studio. Regardless of attachment used, aim for continuous tension throughout the exercise, especially on the way up, where you should control the weight and actively try to resist gravity. Spend quality time getting stronger at lat pull-downs and you may even be able to do pull-ups again!

Pull-Up

The pull-up is a challenging body-weight exercise that targets the upper back muscles, primarily the latissimus dorsi. However, an assisted pull-up machine is the ideal way to learn proper technique without having to lift your entire body weight. This machine was a must-have when I started my gym in 2002 and is a staple exercise for most of my clients. The technique described below will be the same whether using your body weight or an assisted pull-up machine.

INSTRUCTION

- Grasp a pull-up bar with an overhand grip (palms facing away), hands shoulder-width apart or slightly wider. (Note: You do *not* need to use an exceptionally wide grip to "enhance V-taper" or any such nonsense. Some trainees with sketchy shoulders do better with a parallel grip if available.)
- Hang with your arms fully extended but keep tension around your shoulder joint by tensing your shoulder muscles. Think a stretch under tension at the bottom rather than relaxing at the stretch (figure *a*).
- Pull yourself up until your chin is above the bar, squeezing your shoulder blades together at the top of the movement (figure *b*). Either keep your legs stiff and straight or bend at the knee and pull the feet up behind you. Try *not* to swing the legs forward and "kip" to perform your pull-ups. If you have to swing to get up to the bar, go back to assisted pull-ups or lat pull-downs and get stronger.
- Slowly lower yourself back to the starting position.
- Repeat for the desired number of repetitions.

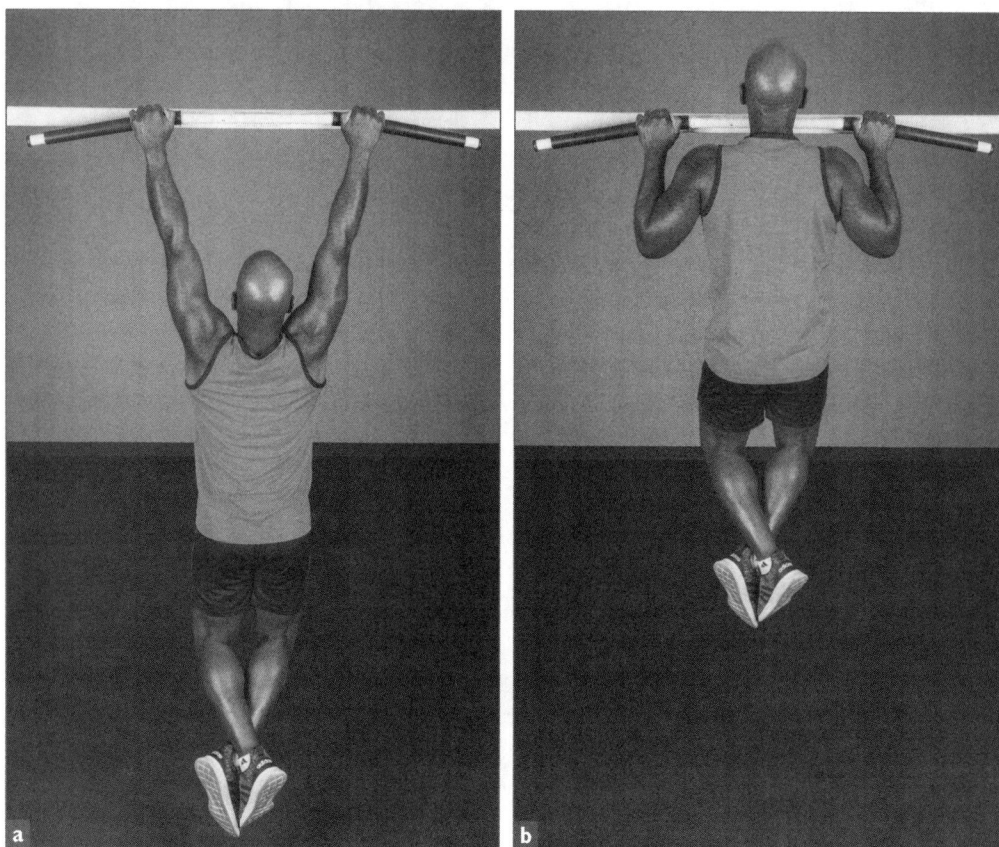

CHAD'S TAKE

Pull-ups are the toughest exercise for most people, regardless of age. Unless you are already quite strong, you will likely need to build strength on the lat pull-down machine or, even better, an assisted pull-up machine, before trying body-weight pull-ups. If not, some trainees use large rubber bands for assistance, although I don't like these nearly as much, and the risk of getting snapped somewhere sensitive is ever present when using bands. In addition to the pronated grip (palms facing away) mentioned above, other variations include a chin-up grip (palms facing you), a parallel or neutral grip (palms facing in) and even a mixed grip (one palm facing you, one palm facing away).

Landmine Row

The landmine row is a compound exercise that targets the middle and upper back muscles. Because of the space-saving nature of the landmine, they are found in many gyms. Myriad attachments are available. For this example we'll use a two-hand grip attachment.

INSTRUCTION

- Place a barbell in a landmine base.
- Stand over the bar with your feet shoulder-width apart and knees slightly bent.
- Grasp the landmine attachment with both hands,
- Bend forward at the hips until your torso is slightly above parallel to the floor
- Lift the weight by extending your hips and knees, keeping your back straight and chest up (figure a).
- Pull the handle or barbell toward your lower chest, keeping your elbows close to your body and squeezing your shoulder blades together at the end of the movement (figure b).
- Slowly lower the weight back down to the starting position.
- Repeat for the desired number of repetitions.

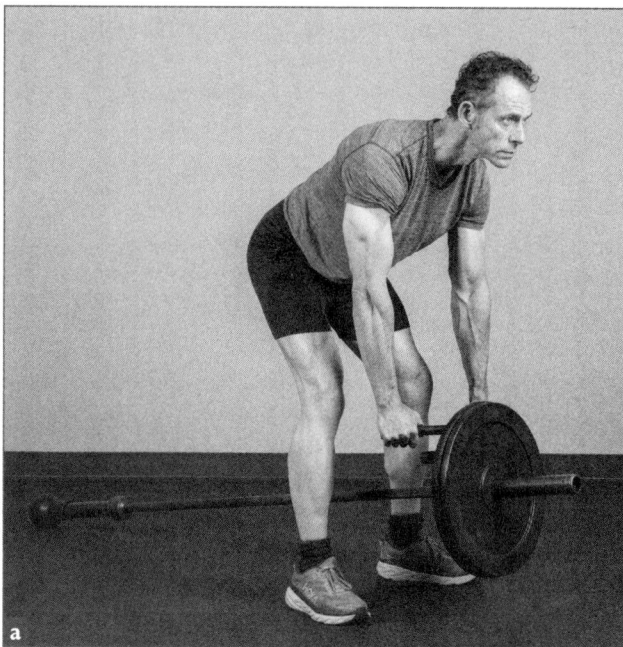

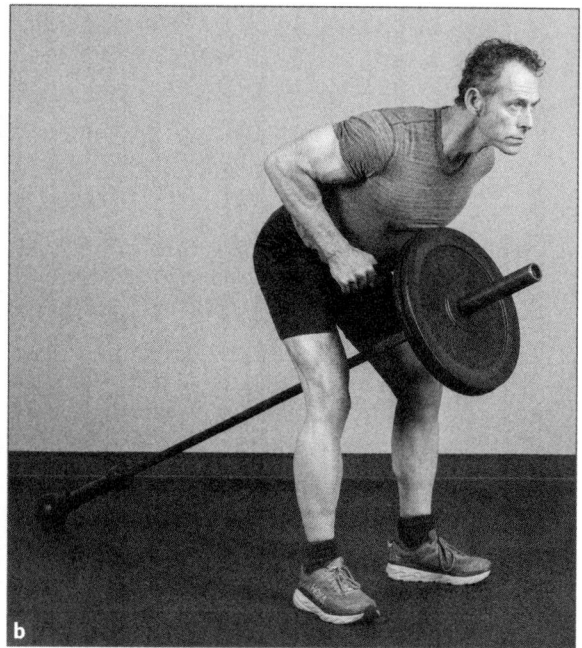

CHAD'S TAKE

There are many different handle attachments for the barbell when using the landmine that allow you to vary the grip used during the row: wide, narrow, straight, parallel, angled, and so on. Try different grips and use what feels most comfortable to you. If available, a chest-supported T-bar row may be a better, safer option than the unsupported landmine variations.

Single-Arm Dumbbell Row on Bench

This unilateral exercise targets the upper and middle back muscles, allowing you to focus on one side at a time. These rows are very useful in gyms that don't have typical rowing machines or cables. Because the hand and knee on the nonworking side are braced on a flat bench, this exercise provides similar benefits to a chest-supported row.

INSTRUCTION

- Place a dumbbell on the floor next to a flat bench.
- Place your right knee and right hand on the bench, with your left foot flat on the floor.
- Grasp the dumbbell with your left hand using an overhand grip (figure *a*).
- Keep your back straight and parallel to the floor.
- Pull the dumbbell toward your lower chest, keeping your elbow close to your body and trying to pull the shoulder blade in toward the spine (figure *b*).
- Slowly lower the dumbbell back down to the starting position.
- Repeat for the desired number of repetitions, then switch sides.

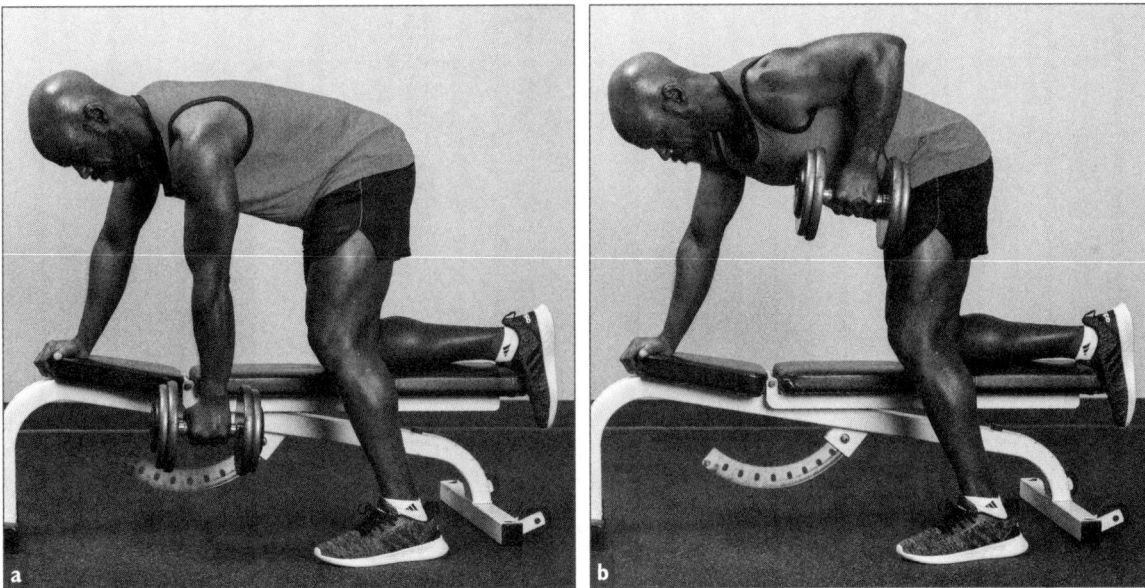

CHAD'S TAKE

While a slight rotation at the hips is OK, avoid using the momentum from overrotating the hip just to use more weight. Keep strict form. Some people like to do this exercise Pendlay style, starting from the ground each rep. I prefer a slight forward to backward arcing motion toward the hip on the pull rather than straight up. Either technique is fine.

Inverted Row

This body-weight exercise targets the upper and middle back muscles. Think of it as a horizontal pull-up. It is *much* more challenging than it first appears. I've also heard this exercise called a *suspended row*, *supine row*, and *horizontal row*. It's all the same thing.

INSTRUCTION

- Adjust suspension straps to a height that allows for a full stretch at the bottom of the movement without hitting the floor.
- Grasp the handles and walk the feet forward and lean back to achieve desired angle with floor (parallel will be the most difficult position) while keeping the hips fully extended and arms straight (figure *a*).
- Pull the upper body up to the handles while keeping your arms at your sides with the wrists in a neutral position, engaging your back muscles, keeping your body in a straight line from head to heels. Your shoulder blades should be pulled together at the top of the movement with the handles at the sides of the pecs (figure *b*).
- Slowly lower yourself back to the starting position.
- Repeat for the desired number of repetitions.

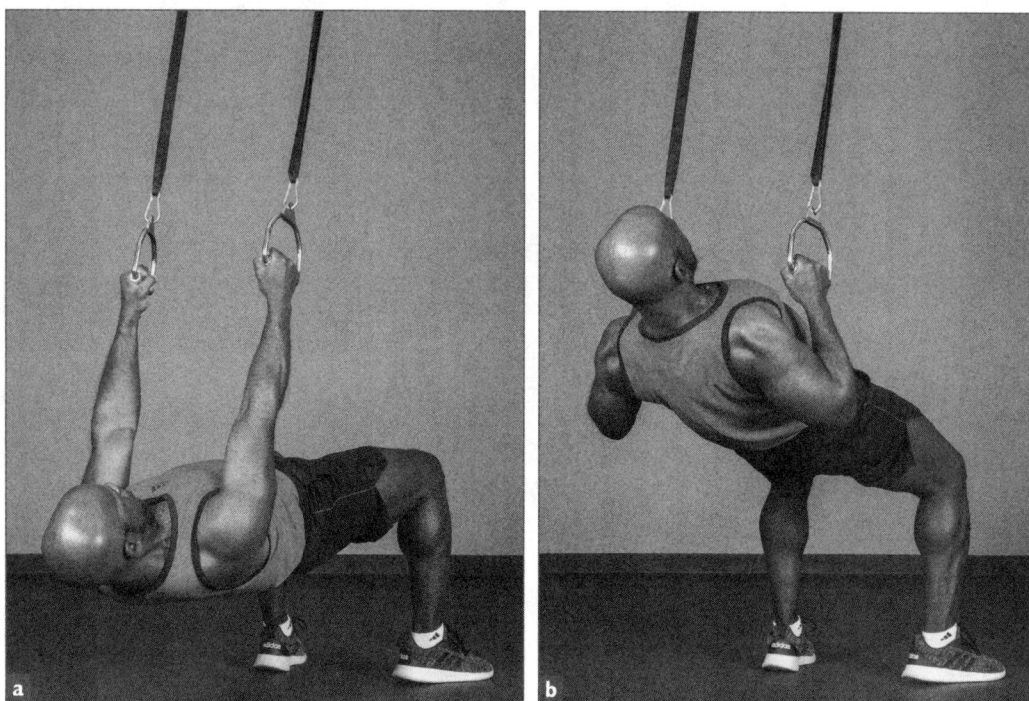

CHAD'S TAKE

I prefer to mirror the same width grip as my bench press. The contraction at the top of the movement helps me to stay tight at the bottom of my bench press. You can also do this exercise using a Smith machine or a barbell in a squat rack if a suspension device is unavailable. Use similar technique and aim for the chest to touch the bar on each rep at roughly nipple level.

Face Pull

This exercise targets the rear deltoids and upper back muscles and is best performed using a cable machine. It is perfectly OK to do these during a shoulder workout rather than a back session. In fact, in the next chapter on shoulders and arms, I recommend a variation that's a bit more specific to the deltoid and rotator cuff called the Cuban-style face pull.

INSTRUCTION

- Adjust the cable pulley to head height and attach a rope handle.
- Grasp the rope handle with both hands using a neutral grip, palms facing each other.
- Step back to create tension in the cable and stand with your feet shoulder-width apart (figure *a*).
- Pull the rope handle toward your face, separating your hands and keeping your elbows high (figure *b*).
- Squeeze your shoulder blades together at the end of the movement.
- Slowly return the rope handle to the starting position, maintaining control throughout the movement.
- Repeat for the desired number of repetitions.

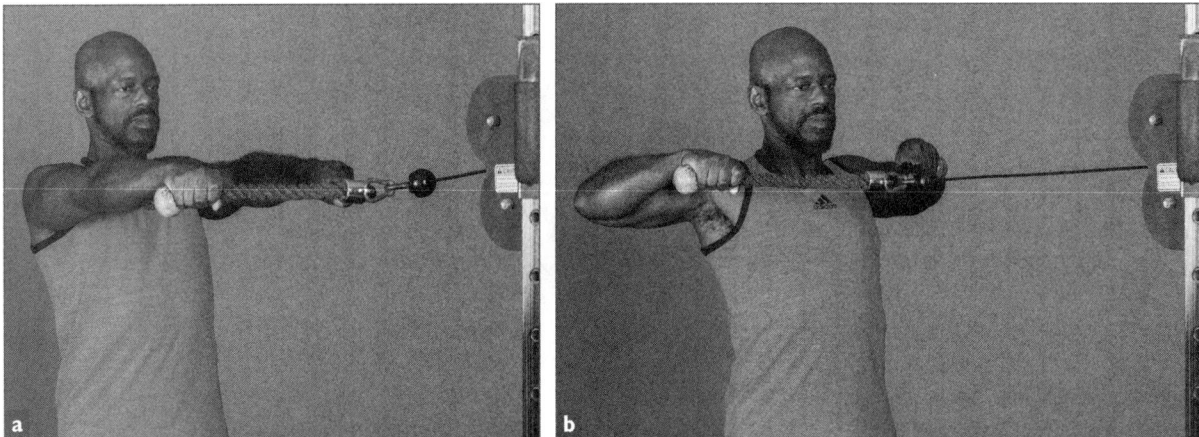

CHAD'S TAKE

Play around with different grips and angles of pull and choose what feels best for you and your shoulders, wrists, and so on. For example, I often use two hand grips on the cable instead of a rope. I'll also lower the pulley slightly if I want to emphasize more back and raise it if I want more shoulders. You could have your palms facing down or slightly adjust the height of your elbows. Also, start light and really get a feel for which muscles are working. It's easy to go too heavy and make this a momentum-filled movement.

Seated Cable Row

The seated cable row targets the latissimus dorsi and upper back muscles and is similar to the landmine and machine rows but typically without the chest support.

INSTRUCTION

- Most seated row machines are fixed with no seat or footplate adjustments available. If adjustments are available, make sure you have room to sit upright with your legs in front of you with a slight bend and can lean forward in the stretch without hitting the weight stack.

- Attach the desired grip handle to the cable pulley. (As with pull-downs, you have many handle options for this exercise. Use what is most comfortable for you and allows you to feel the muscles being worked.)

- Sit with your feet against the footplate (if available), knees slightly bent, and grasp the handle.

- Sit upright with your chest up and shoulders back, maintaining a slight arch in your lower back (figure a).

- Pull the handle toward your lower chest, keeping your elbows out to the sides and squeezing your shoulder blades together at the end of the movement, attempting to bring the handle to the abdomen (figure b).

- Slowly return the handle to the starting position.

- Repeat for the desired number of repetitions.

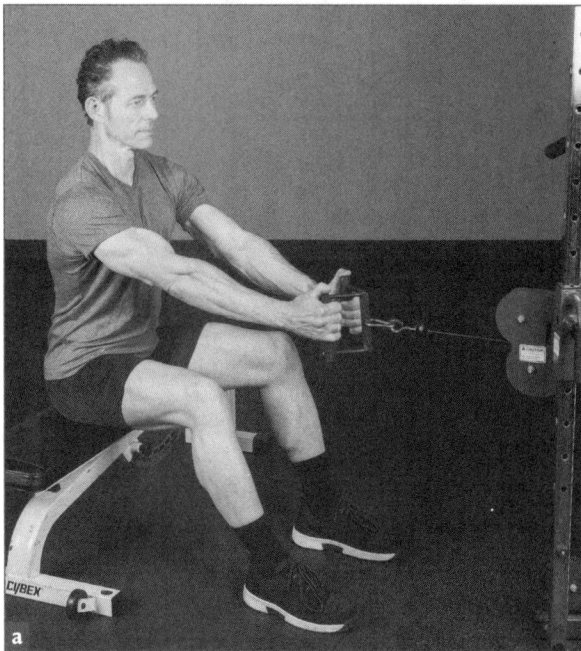 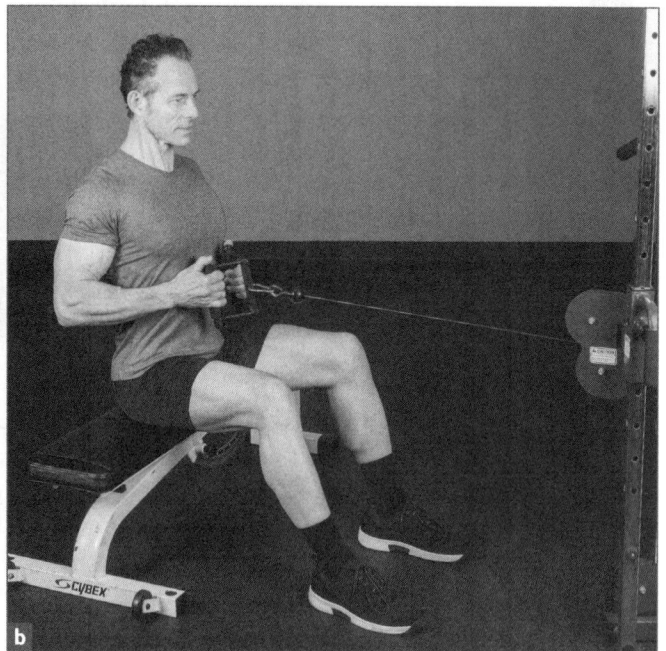

CHAD'S TAKE

As with the machine row, begin the motion by drawing back the shoulders without bending the elbows. Also, take care not to lean back too far with the lower back and use momentum. This is more common here since there is no chest support. I think we 50-somethings should opt for a chest-supported row, especially with a history of lower back issues. If you only have access to a cable row machine, be sure to maintain strict form and don't lift any weight so heavy you cannot maintain this form.

CHAPTER 7

Shoulders, Biceps, and Triceps

Nothing indicates to the rest of the world that you train quite like a nice set of shoulders and arms. And ask anyone from age 5 to 95 to "make a muscle" and they'll automatically hit a biceps pose. There's even an emoji for it!

Unfortunately, a lot of folks over the age of 50 are unhappy with how their arms and shoulders look, and many no longer feel confident wearing sleeveless shirts. We are about to change that! So if you want arms like Arnold or Linda Hamilton in *Terminator 2*, the exercises in this chapter will target the shoulders, biceps, and triceps and ensure that you achieve balance, symmetry, and overall upper-body strength.

But while looking good is great, we also need to be strong. Case in point, there's a shoulder exercise called the overhead press that I nicknamed the "overhead bin exercise." Why? Because if you have to stow your carry-on bag in an airplane's overhead bin, you'd better be able to lift 35 pounds (U.S. carry-on weight limit) over your head unless you want to be dependent on others when you travel.

For years now I've seen the overhead press on numerous "5 exercises you should never do over age 50" type articles and blog posts, as if there is something inherently dangerous about doing this exercise after 50. Their rationale is it's "hard" on the shoulder and rotator cuff muscles, which I'd counter is precisely the reason you should be overhead pressing. When it comes to strength and flexibility, the adage "use it or lose it" couldn't be truer.

Unless you want to lose the ability to use a shelf higher than your head, or you don't want to access the overhead bin when you travel, you need to overhead press. And while I would never encourage someone to go against a doctor's advice, multiple older clients of mine have had physicians tell them things like they would "never have full use of their hand again" or should "never lift more than 5 or 10 pounds again" but proved those limitations wrong with proper rehab and training. So, listen to your doctor, but also be your own advocate.

Many trainees do too many direct arm exercises, especially biceps. The triceps and biceps are relatively small muscles and get a healthy dose of work by assisting during many chest and back exercises. So while a little direct arm work is fine, endless sets of multiple curling variations, for example, are simply unnecessary—although they are fun to do!

Remember that proper form and technique are essential for maximizing muscle growth and minimizing the risk of injury, so pay close attention to the descriptions provided.

SHOULDER EXERCISES

The shoulder is a complex joint that is responsible for a wide range of movements. While technically a ball-and-socket joint like the hips, the shoulders have a very shallow socket, therefore it's critical to have strong *deltoids* (anterior, medial, and posterior) to improve shoulder stability and enhance upper-body performance.

Most people will find shoulder exercises like overhead pressing and lateral raises to be more comfortable if done in what is called the *scapular plane* as opposed to the *frontal plane*, which we might normally think of with those exercises. The scapular plane is about 30 to 45 degrees in front of the body because of the motion of the scapula as it moves around our rounded rib cage. So if we keep our arms at this angle while doing lateral raises or presses, we can get proper motion around the shoulder with less chance of shoulder impingement pain. That being said, I tend to do my overhead pressing in the frontal plane. By keeping my arms back, I feel better tension on my deltoids through the press. I do typically do my lateral raises in the scapular plane, however. Feel free to experiment, but if you have any preexisting shoulder pain, or a random pain flares up, stick to the scapular plane.

As with the arms, many trainees do too many shoulder exercises. They do overhead presses and lateral raises and rear delt flys and front raises, all in the same workout. But these muscles are relatively small and, like arms, get a lot of work during chest and back exercises, so I encourage you to go easy on the amount of direct deltoid work.

For example, I almost never program direct anterior deltoid exercises (e.g., front raises), because the front delts work very hard on bench-pressing exercises, and I find direct work unnecessary. In fact, as my own bench press grew to over 300 pounds, my anterior deltoids got extremely well developed with zero direct anterior deltoid exercises. That's not to say front raises aren't beneficial for someone lacking anterior deltoid development, but for most trainees who already hit chest exercises hard, the exercise is superfluous.

You might then think that direct posterior deltoid work is unnecessary, too, as the posterior deltoids are worked during pulling exercises for the upper back. And while this is true, it's still good to give them a little direct work along with the muscles of the rotator cuff that externally rotate the shoulder. I actually think specific rotator cuff work is more important than direct rear delt exercises—so important, in fact, that I've included a sidebar to dig deeper into how to strengthen our rotators to help "bulletproof" our aging shoulders.

Rotator Cuff

You have probably heard of the rotator cuff, or more likely about injuries to the rotator cuff. Rotator cuff injuries are common in overhead athletes such as pitchers and volleyball players. But you may not know exactly what the rotator cuff is, why it's important, or how to strengthen it.

The rotator cuff is not one thing, it's four things—four muscles, that is. They are relatively small, especially compared to the large muscles in the rest of this book, but they are some of the most important muscles of the body, especially for the older trainee.

The rotator cuff is made up of the *supraspinatus*, *infraspinatus*, *teres minor*, and *subscapularis* muscles. While these are not muscles you'll be flexing in the mirror, they are critical to the health and function of the shoulder girdle and can be a limiting factor in working the bigger show muscles if they aren't strong.

The muscles of the rotator cuff all arise from the shoulder blade and attach to the upper arm bone, just from different positions and angles. Suffice it to say that these muscles are important stabilizers in nearly every type of shoulder movement. They keep the upper end of your upper arm bone in the proper place as you move your arm in any direction.

You might wonder that since these muscles are working on nearly every upper-body exercise, and because they are so small, do you really need to directly target them? Yes and no. First, if you have a rotator cuff strain or tear, you'll likely be prescribed rotator cuff exercises as part of your therapy. But even if your shoulders are fine, you still may want to do a little direct work for the muscles of the rotator cuff that do external rotation, the infraspinatus and the teres minor. Why just these two?

Think back to when you first started lifting weights. Were you concerned about looking like a hunched-forward bodybuilder? Well, that hunch is caused by too much internal rotation of the shoulder, culminating in an ape-like look.

Several muscles contribute to internal rotation, especially the pec major. But it might surprise you to know that the lats, those big back muscles, help to internally rotate the shoulder. Also, the subscapularis of the rotator cuff internally rotates the shoulder, so, barring injury to the subscapularis requiring rehab, I don't believe extra internal rotation work is productive, especially when your pecs and lats are already doing so much to hunch you forward.

I like to think of the muscles around the shoulder as guy wires helping to keep the shoulders in place. And our small external rotators (infraspinatus and teres minor) have to counteract those big pecs and lats to keep the arm bones in the right place while we move. Everyone can benefit from some direct external rotation work, but I find it critical for those of us who do a lot of heavy chest and lat work.

Fortunately, it's pretty easy to do external rotation exercise, and many tools—from a dumbbell or cables to bands or tubing—can do the job well. My favorites are cable exercises for their ability to keep continuous, consistent tension on the muscles throughout the range of motion. Elastic resistance is another good option; however, the tension changes throughout the range of motion and you never know exactly how much resistance you're using, so you have to go by "feel." Dumbbells are OK, but again, the resistance will feel different depending on where you are in the range of motion because of the effects of gravity.

These are my three favorite external rotation exercises, one using cables, one using elastic resistance (rubber band or tubing), and one using a dumbbell.

(continued)

Rotator Cuff   *(continued)*

Cable External Rotation

- Set the cable pulley to elbow height and attach a single handle.
- Stand perpendicular to the cable machine, holding the handle with the arm furthest from the machine (figure 7.1a).
- Keep your elbow bent at 90 degrees and tucked against your side.
- Start with your hand near your stomach, and rotate your arm outward until your forearm is almost perpendicular to your torso (figure 7.1b).
- Maintain control as you slowly return to the starting position. Do not allow the weight stack to touch between reps.
- Keep your shoulder down and avoid shrugging or twisting your torso.

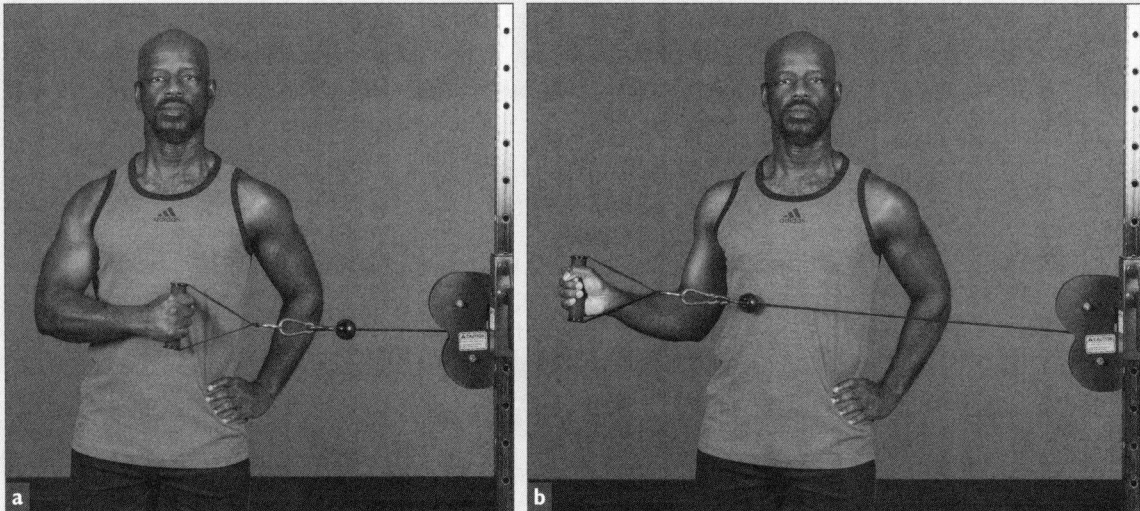

FIGURE 7.1   External rotation exercises for the rotator cuff: cable external rotation.

Band Ws

- Hold one end of an elastic exercise band or tubing in each hand.
- Stand tall with your elbows bent at 90 degrees and positioned near your sides (figure 7.2a).
- Rotate your forearms outward while squeezing your shoulder blades together, forming a W with your arms (figure 7.2b).
- Hold the contraction briefly, then return to the starting position with control. Try to keep a bit of tension at the front and not completely relax between reps.
- Keep your posture upright and avoid excessive arching in your lower back.

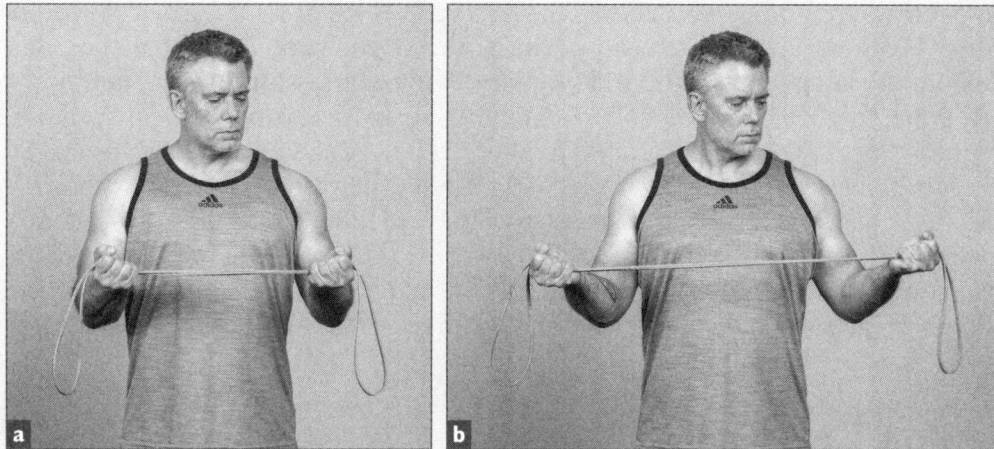

FIGURE 7.2   External rotation exercises for the rotator cuff: band Ws.

Dumbbell External Rotation (Elbow on Knee)

- Sit sideways on a bench with one foot flat on the floor and the other foot on the bench with the knee bent at about a 45-degree angle. Rest that elbow on the top of your knee just inside the kneecap.

- Hold a dumbbell with a palm-down grip, keeping your elbow bent at 90 degrees (figure 7.3a).

- Start with the dumbbell hanging down, then externally rotate your arm by lifting the weight outward and upward (figure 7.3b).

- Pause briefly at the top, then lower the dumbbell back to the starting position in a controlled manner.

- Avoid using momentum, and keep the movement slow and controlled.

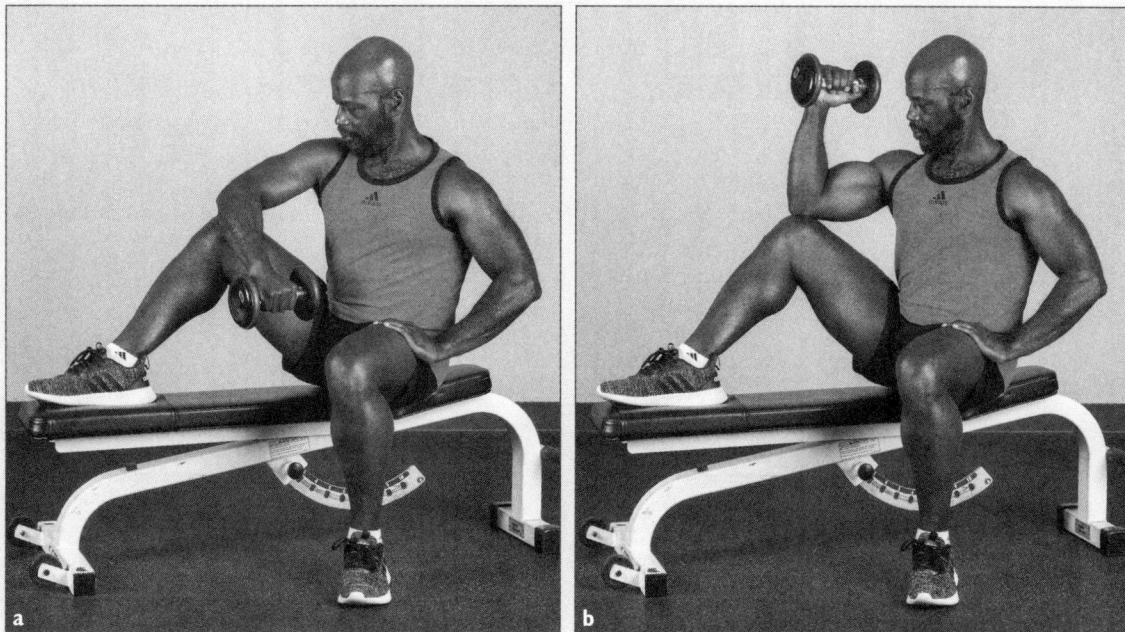

FIGURE 7.3   External rotation exercises for the rotator cuff: dumbbell external rotation (elbow on knee).

As I mentioned, if you want to be able to lift your suitcase into and out of an overhead bin on an airplane or use the top shelves of your cupboard, you'd better be strong in the overhead position. But if you didn't pass the shoulder flexion test in chapter 4, you'll do better overhead pressing using a landmine setup than barbells or dumbbells. Remember, if we have proper mobility in our shoulder joints, we should be able to overhead press, with our arms vertical at the top of the movement (basically aligned with the ears), but without arching the lower back and raising the rib cage (called "rib flare"). One thing I like about the landmine press is that you can lean forward slightly in the top position and stretch out those tight tissues restricting shoulder flexion. I've had countless clients progress to overhead pressing with free weights after just a short time working with the landmine.

Seated Dumbbell Shoulder Press

If I could only do one "vertical press" exercise, it would be this one. Two things make it of particular value to the over-50 crowd: First, since you are seated, you won't be able to use any momentum from leg drive that might tempt you to use weights that are too heavy. Second, since using dumbbells means the left and right sides move independently, you can make subtle adjustments to wrist and elbow positioning and work around any aches or pains in those joints.

INSTRUCTION

- Sit on a bench with back support and hold a dumbbell in each hand at shoulder level, palms facing forward (figure *a*).
- Press the dumbbells up until your arms are fully extended above your head (figure *b*).
- Slowly lower the weights back to the starting position and repeat.

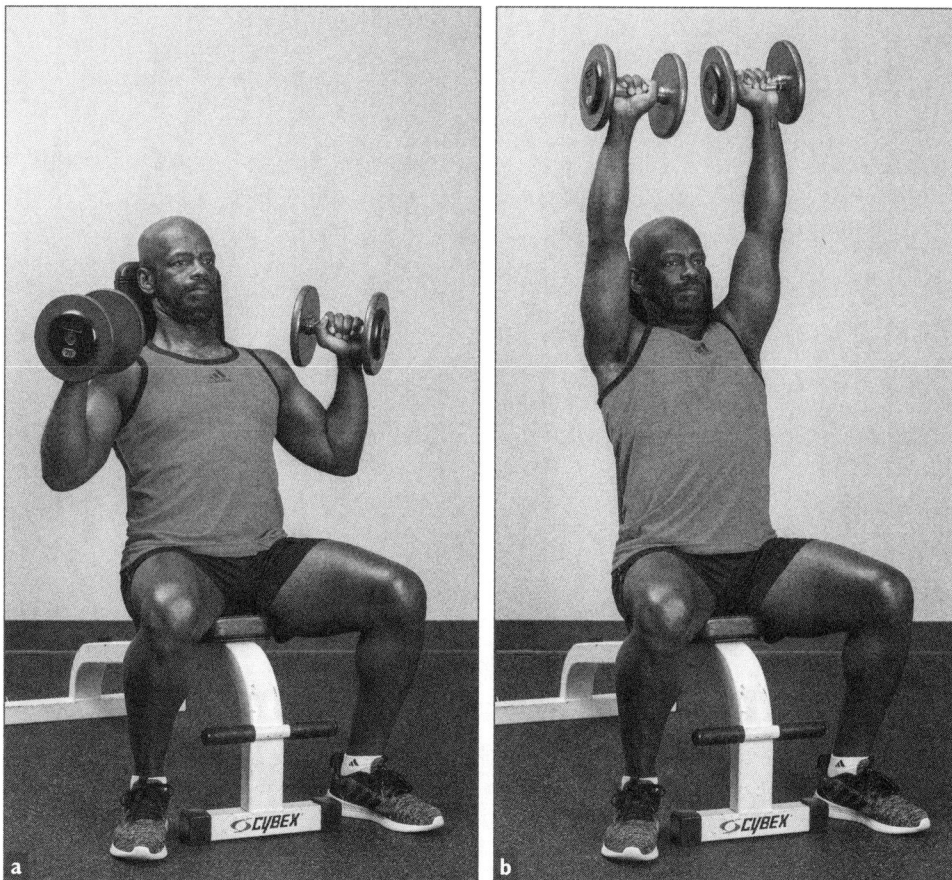

CHAD'S TAKE

Trainees with healthy shoulders will likely feel better tension and connection to the deltoids when pressing in the palms-forward position. However, many will find they feel pain or even clicking when pressing in this position. Most of my clients with this issue can overhead press without these complaints simply by allowing the elbows to start in a more forward position (scapular plane) and keeping a neutral grip (palms facing in) on the dumbbells throughout the movement.

Standing Barbell Military Press

This old-school exercise is the granddaddy of vertical presses. You can push heavy weights and put size on the deltoids and triceps pretty handily. I still prefer overhead pressing with dumbbells over a barbell, but if you don't have access to heavier dumbbells, this exercise could be for you.

INSTRUCTION

- Stand with feet shoulder-width apart and grasp a barbell with a grip slightly wider than shoulder-width, palms facing away from you (usually done in a power rack).
- Position the barbell at collarbone level (figure *a*).
- Press the barbell upward until your arms are fully extended above your head (figure *b*).
- Slowly lower the bar back to collarbone level and repeat.

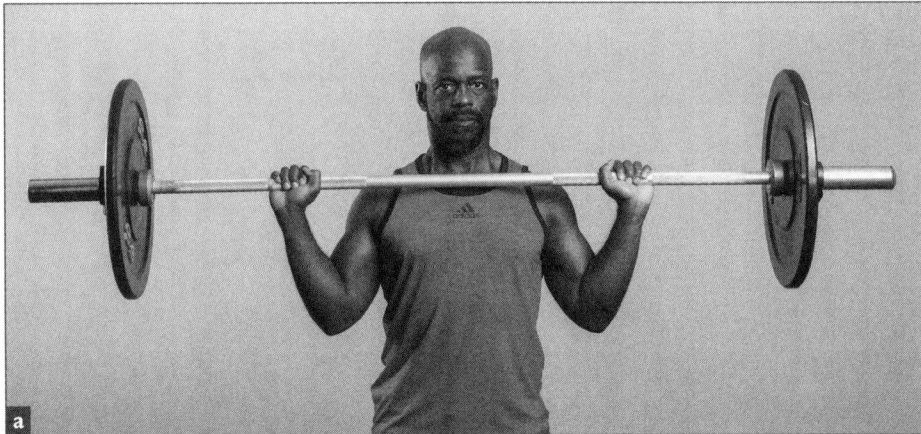

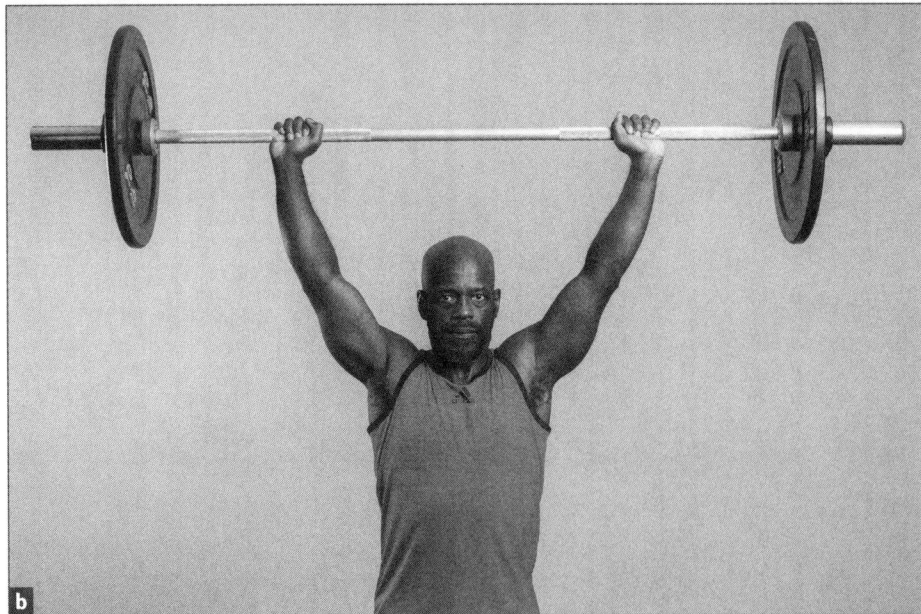

CHAD'S TAKE

I do these exercises in my own training but rarely with clients. I find dumbbells or the landmine machine easier for newer clients to learn, and much safer for older trainees with "irritable" shoulders. Be aware that if you have any preexisting shoulder issues, you could feel pain doing these and may even lack the necessary range of motion to do them properly. If that's the case, use that barbell as a landmine instead, or use dumbbells and avoid strict barbell military pressing.

In years past, the behind-the-neck press was a training staple, but unless you have strong and healthy shoulders already, it's probably best to leave this version in the past. You could do these seated in a rack with an adjustable bench at near vertical. This is a great way to ensure you aren't using your lower body too much and keep the focus on your shoulders and triceps.

Single-Arm Cable Lateral Raise

You might be more familiar with the dumbbell lateral raise to work the medial deltoids, but I prefer cables. If you don't have a cable set-up where you train, feel free to use dumbbells (usually both arms simultaneously) instead.

INSTRUCTION

- Set a low cable pulley at hip height or lower. Stand with feet shoulder-width apart, with your side to the cable pulley while holding a cable with a single handle in the opposite hand (cable crosses in front of body) (figure *a*).
- With a bend in your elbow, raise your arm out to the side and slightly to the front of the body until it is parallel to the floor (figure *b*).
- Slowly lower your arm back to the starting position and repeat.
- Switch sides and repeat.

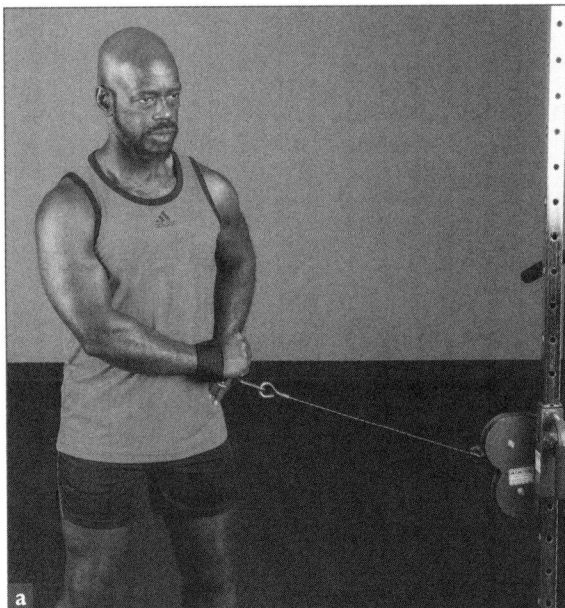

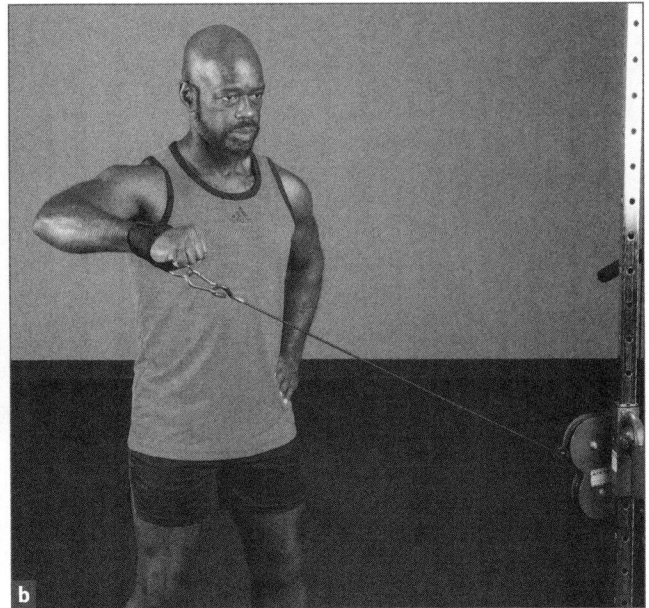

CHAD'S TAKE

I much prefer using cables for this exercise since they allow for continuous tension on the deltoids throughout the range of motion, which dumbbells don't because of the limitations of gravity. I especially like using a hook-and-loop attachment around the wrist to connect the cables. With that, you don't have to worry about gripping a handle and can instead focus on the deltoids. These attachments also eliminate the wrist pain some people feel when using regular single handles. Also, it can be beneficial to lean forward with the chest supported by a bench or simply do the exercise while seated to avoid unconscious momentum from your body especially when trying to lift too heavy on this exercise.

Seated Bent-Over Dumbbell Rear Delt Fly

This is a great free-weight version of a rear delt fly. Take care to ensure the elbows are kept at close to a 90-degree angle from the body. If you allow the elbows to drop close to the sides of the body, you'll be able to go heavier, but it's because the back muscles will take over more of the work than the rear delts. Keep the weight lighter and the form tighter.

INSTRUCTION

- Sit on the end of a flat bench. Bend at the hips, keeping your back straight. Hold a dumbbell in each hand (figure *a*).
- With a slight bend in your elbows, raise your arms out to the sides, squeezing your shoulder blades together (figure *b*).
- Slowly lower your arms back to the starting position and repeat.

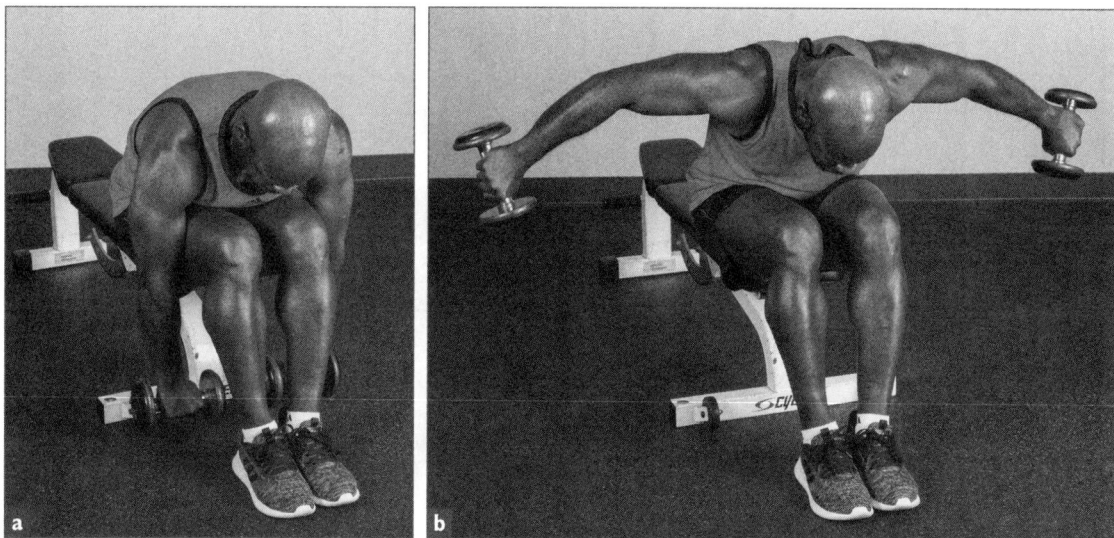

CHAD'S TAKE

I still prefer to do rear flys on the pec deck or the cable crossovers because of the continuous tension they provide. However, if your gym is limited, using dumbbells is fine; it's just a mildly uncomfortable position for some people. If an adjustable incline bench is available, try this face down on about a 30- to 45-degree angle. That can be more comfortable than leaning forward.

Cable Upright Row

This old-school exercise fell out of favor for several years because of fear of shoulder joint impingement. I've found that as long as you don't raise the elbows much above shoulder level, impingement probably won't be an issue, but be aware that many people find the wrist position at the top of the movement to be uncomfortable if not painful.

INSTRUCTION

- Stand with feet shoulder-width apart and grasp an EZ-curl attachment on a low cable pulley with a close grip, palms facing your body at arm's length in front of you (figure a). Ensure that the pulley is set low enough that the weight stack is not touching in the start position.
- Pull the weight upward, leading with your elbows and keeping the attachment close to your body until it reaches chest level (figure b).
- Slowly lower the weight back to the starting position and repeat.

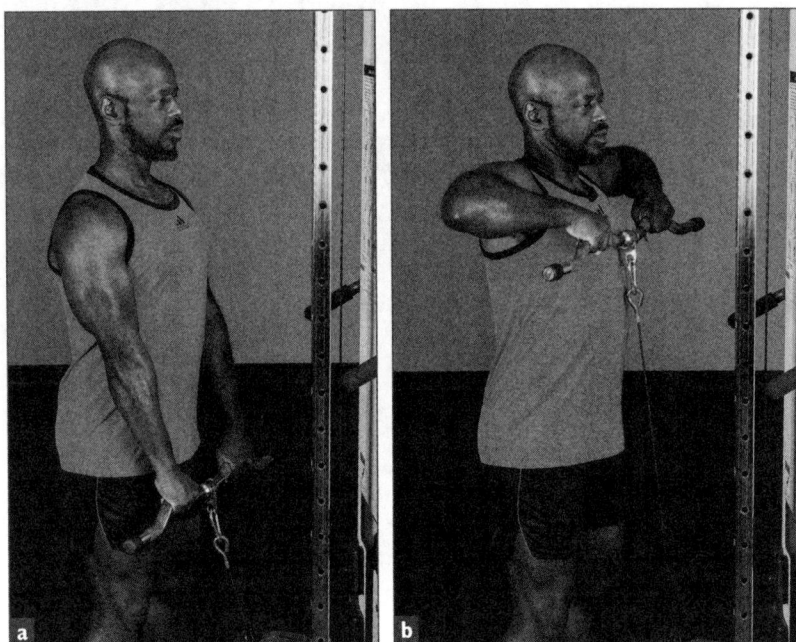

CHAD'S TAKE

I prefer to perform upright rows with an EZ-bar attachment on a cable machine, but a free-weight version with dumbbells or an EZ-curl bar is a viable alternative. I don't find straight bar attachments to be as comfortable as the EZ-bar attachment. Some people like to use a rope for these. If you can't find a comfortable way to do these for both the shoulders and the wrists, I recommend using other exercises for shoulder development.

Dumbbell Seesaw Press

This overhead pressing variation provides a bonus to the core in the frontal plane because of the bracing you do while pressing up on only one side and resisting the urge to laterally flex the spine (lean over).

INSTRUCTION

- Stand with feet shoulder-width apart. Hold a dumbbell in each hand at shoulder level, palms facing forward (or in, if preferred). Press the dominant arm overhead so one arm is at shoulder level and one is overhead (figure *a*).
- Simultaneously press the nondominant arm overhead while lowering the dominant arm to shoulder level (figure *b*).
- Repeat the motion to return to the start position and complete one repetition. Repeat for desired number of reps.

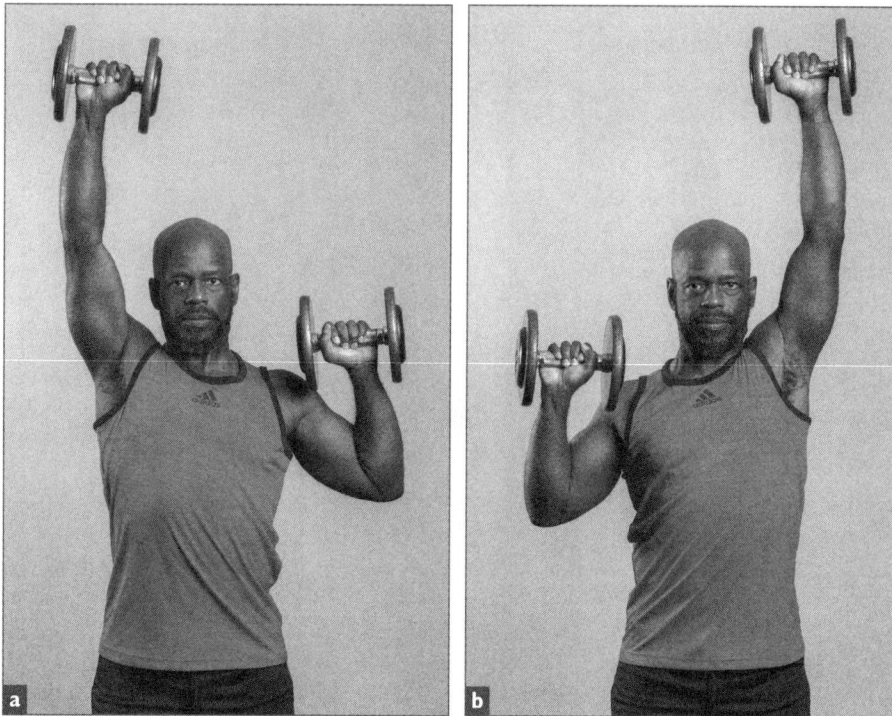

CHAD'S TAKE

I love the challenge to strength, coordination, and stability provided by this exercise, all pluses for those of us over 50. Take care not to lean side to side when pressing but rather brace and stabilize with the core. I especially like these if you have only lighter dumbbells available or if you have existing shoulder issues, as they provide more of a challenge with lighter weights than traditional overhead dumbbell presses.

Cuban-Style Face Pull

What makes it "Cuban" (don't ask me why) is the external rotation during the exercise. Where the rope face pull maintains a constant external rotation as you pull the rope to your body, the Cuban starts with arms straight out in front of you, and then as you draw the elbows back in alignment with the shoulders, you'll perform an external rotation of the shoulders.

INSTRUCTION

- Attach two hand grips to a cable machine at face level.
- Stand with feet shoulder-width apart and grasp the handles with a pronated, palms-down grip, arms extended in front of you (figure *a*).
- Pull the handles toward your face, keeping your elbows high (figure *b*). When the elbows align with the shoulders, externally rotate the arms until they end up in an L position while squeezing your shoulder blades together (figure *c*).
- Slowly extend your arms back to the starting position and repeat.

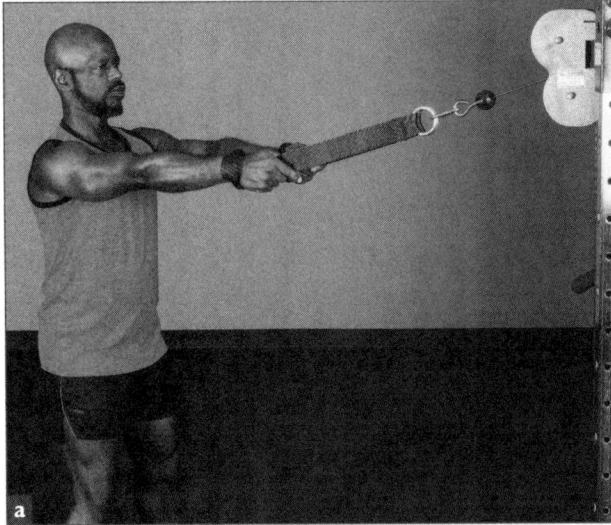

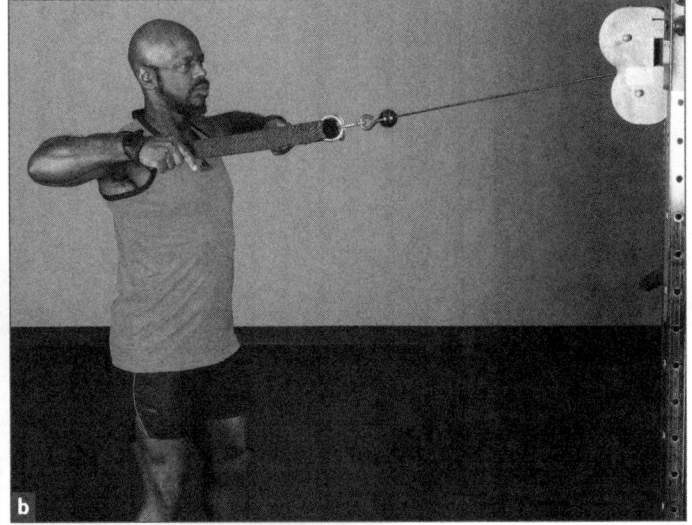

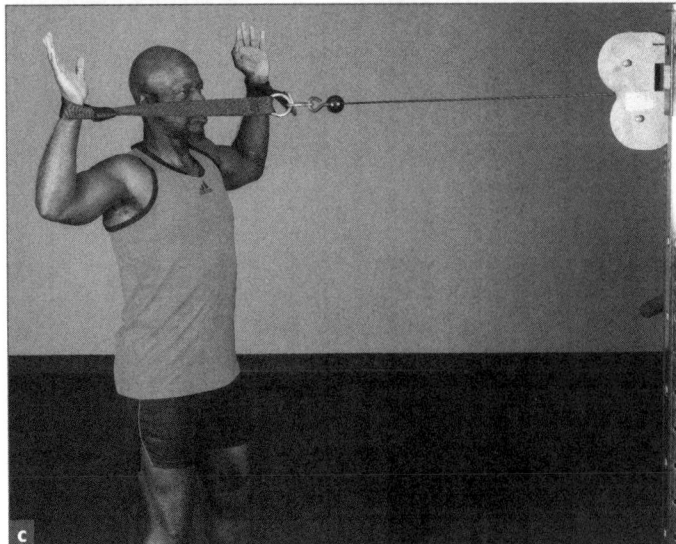

CHAD'S TAKE

I love this exercise! It targets the rotator cuff muscles more than the regular face pulls described in chapter 6. I have a unique attachment from Spud Inc. that has two long looping straps. This allows me to anchor the weight at my wrists rather than holding onto a rope. Highly recommended! All the face-pull variations are great options to keep our battered shoulders healthy and strong as we get older.

Single-Arm Landmine Press

This is my go-to overhead press for those whose range of motion is limited and who can't lift their arms straight overhead in line with their ears (see shoulder flexion test in chapter 4). Even if you can pass the shoulder flexion test, the landmine press is still a great alternative to keep in the rotation.

INSTRUCTION

- Secure one end of a barbell into a landmine attachment. If you don't have a landmine attachment, position the end of the barbell securely into a corner of the room (ensure that it won't slip or damage the wall).
- Stand facing the barbell and pick up the free end. Your feet should be staggered and shoulder-width apart for a solid base.
- Bring the barbell up to shoulder height, holding the end of the barbell in your hand (palm forward), and the elbow of the arm holding the barbell bent and close to your body (figure *a*).
- Engage your core and keep your spine neutral as you press the barbell upward until your arm is fully extended (figure *b*).
- Repeat for the desired number of repetitions, then switch arms.

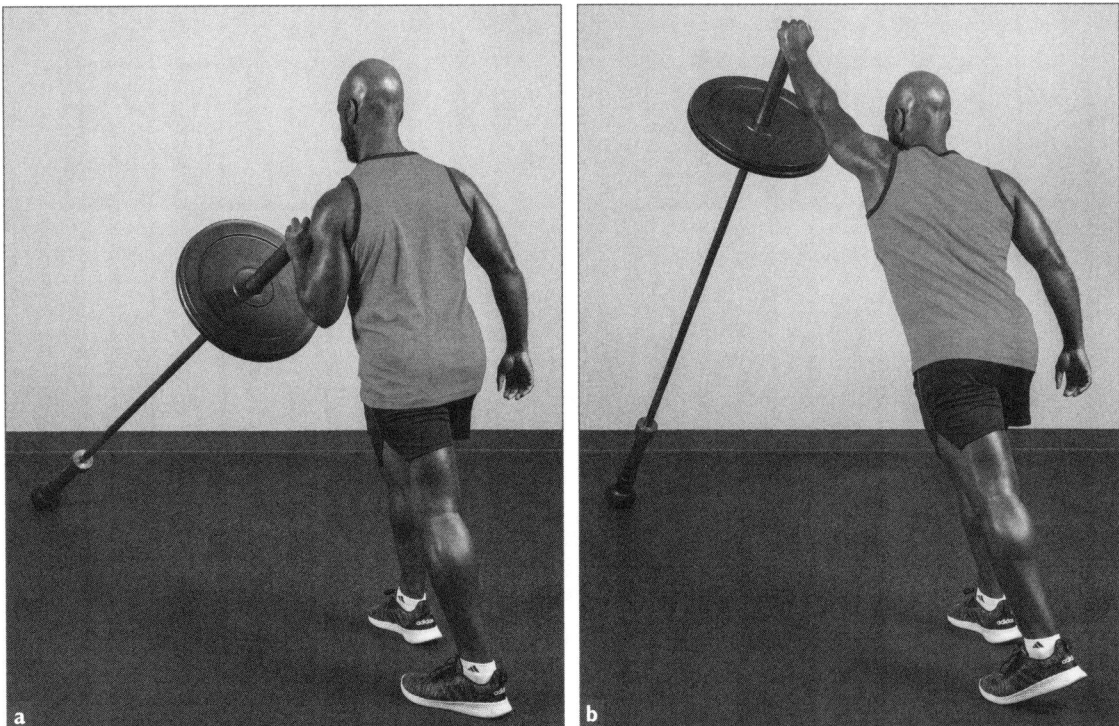

CHAD'S TAKE

There are many single-arm and two-arm attachments for landmine presses. While you can just place the end of the barbell in the palm of your hand, I find attachments to be a safer, cleaner alternative. You can also play around with pressing from the half-kneeling position (one knee down, preferably on an Airex pad or similar) or a high kneel position (both knees on Airex with legs in a "tall," hip-extended position). You'll naturally need to go a bit lighter with kneeling variations because the positioning makes unconscious assistance from your body less likely.

Seated Machine Rear Delt Fly

This exercise is typically done facing in on a pec deck machine, though some brands do make dedicated rear delt fly machines. If you have well-developed rear delts from back exercises, you can probably leave these out, but I like to keep them in the rotation myself.

INSTRUCTION

- Sit facing the machine with your chest against the pad and grasp the handles (figure *a*). (Depending on the brand of machine, the handles may have the palms facing in or down. Do what is most comfortable for you.)
- With a slight bend in your elbows, pull the handles out to the sides, squeezing your shoulder blades together (figure *b*).
- Slowly return to the starting position, but avoid touching the weight stack between reps. Repeat.

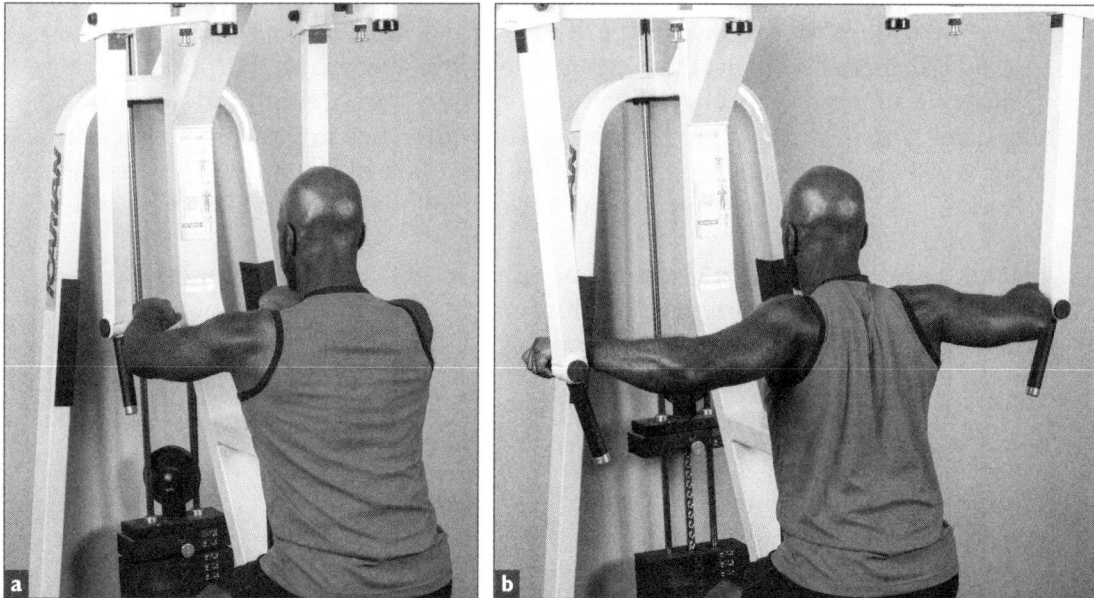

CHAD'S TAKE

If you have a pec deck or rear delt fly machine, it will likely be easier to learn and use regularly than bent-over dumbbell or cable variations of rear delt flys. If you don't have one available, instead focus on face pulls (regular and Cuban variations) as well as the external rotator cuff exercises earlier in this chapter. If we want to keep our over-50 shoulders healthy, we need to do at least a little rear delt or external rotator work.

BICEPS EXERCISES

The *biceps brachii* is a two-headed muscle responsible for supinating the fore-arm and assisting the brachialis muscle in flexing the elbow. In actuality, biceps exercises are just as much if not more so brachialis exercises. For our purposes, consider both muscles worked unless otherwise stated.

Strengthening the biceps and brachialis will improve grip strength and upper-arm aesthetics. But the truth is most biceps exercises are redundant. The muscles themselves are fairly small and take very little stimulus to be worked properly. There is simply no need to do two, three, or four variations of biceps curls in a workout. Pick one, work hard, and move on.

Now let's talk grip strength. Several studies have shown a positive relationship between grip strength and successful aging. People with lower levels of grip strength have a higher incidence of cardiovascular disease, respiratory disease, cancer, and all-cause mortality (Celis-Morales et al. 2015; Cooper, Kuh, and Hardy 2010; Leong et al. 2015). However, I don't believe this means we need to devote time to specific exercises like hand grippers or ball squeezes, although you can certainly do these if you like them. More research is needed, but it's possible that it's not grip strength itself, but rather the overall physical strength and well-being associated with a stronger grip that makes the difference in health outcomes. In other words, if your grip is strong, the rest of you is likely strong too. Testing grip strength is simply an easy way to screen a lot of people quickly for overall well-being.

I don't do direct grip work, nor do I program specific grip work for my clients. I find that people's grip strength will improve along with the rest of their body as they continue to progress in their training with heavier and heavier weights.

Dumbbell Hammer Curl

The dumbbell hammer curl is the first curling exercise I teach clients. Its name comes from the neutral position the wrist is kept in while you curl—like holding a hammer. I prefer to start clients with dumbbells because it will elucidate any strength differences between the right and left sides better than a barbell.

INSTRUCTION

- Stand with feet shoulder-width apart and hold a dumbbell in each hand, hands at your sides, palms facing your thighs (figure *a*).
- Curl the dumbbells toward your shoulders, keeping your palms facing each other. A cue I use is to have the dumbbells "frame the pecs" at the top, so the weight on the top end of the dumbbell is above the pecs and the weight on the bottom is below. If you curl so high you can see the bottom side of the dumbbell in the mirror, your elbow has come forward and you've curled too high (figure *b*).
- Slowly lower the dumbbells back to the starting position and repeat.

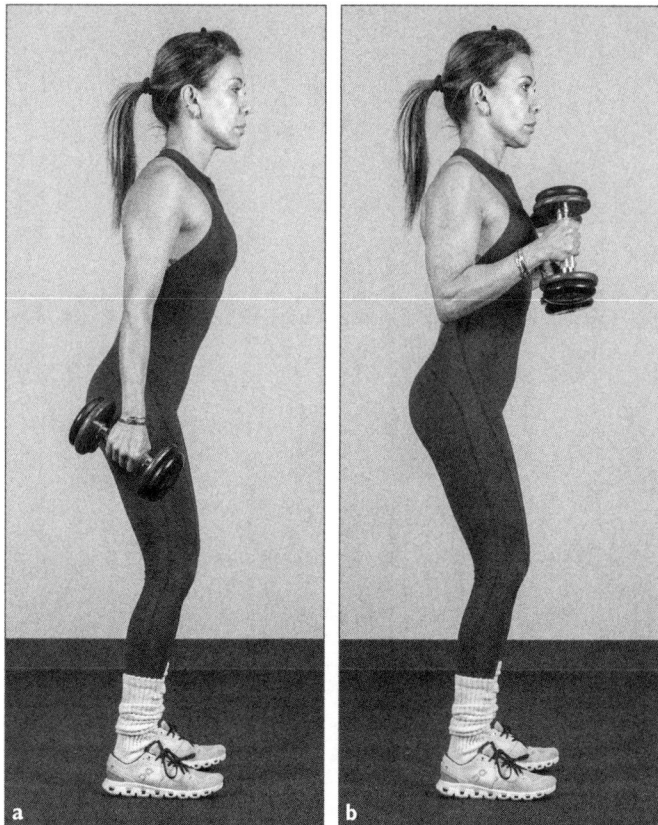

CHAD'S TAKE

The dumbbell hammer curl is my favorite form of curl. It focuses a bit more on the brachialis muscle underlying the biceps since you are not supinating the wrist during the curl. The brachialis is the prime flexor of the elbow and sits underneath the biceps. A well-developed brachialis is more important to upper-arm development than the biceps is, in my opinion. Once you've mastered it, you can try supinating the wrist on the way up instead of maintaining the hammer position. This will add a bit more biceps stimulus.

Standing EZ-Bar Curl

Historically, the straight barbell curl has been *the* biceps exercise. But I prefer using an EZ-curl bar or dumbbells instead of a straight bar because of the more comfortable wrist position. If you don't have access to an EZ-curl bar and your wrists are flexible enough, you can use the straight bar to curl using the same technique.

INSTRUCTION

- Stand with the feet shoulder-width apart and grasp an EZ-curl bar with an underhand but slightly pronated grip. Most EZ bars will have a wide and narrow grip option for this wrist position (figure *a*).
- Curl the barbell toward your chest, keeping your elbows stationary (figure *b*).
- Slowly lower the EZ bar back to the starting position and repeat.

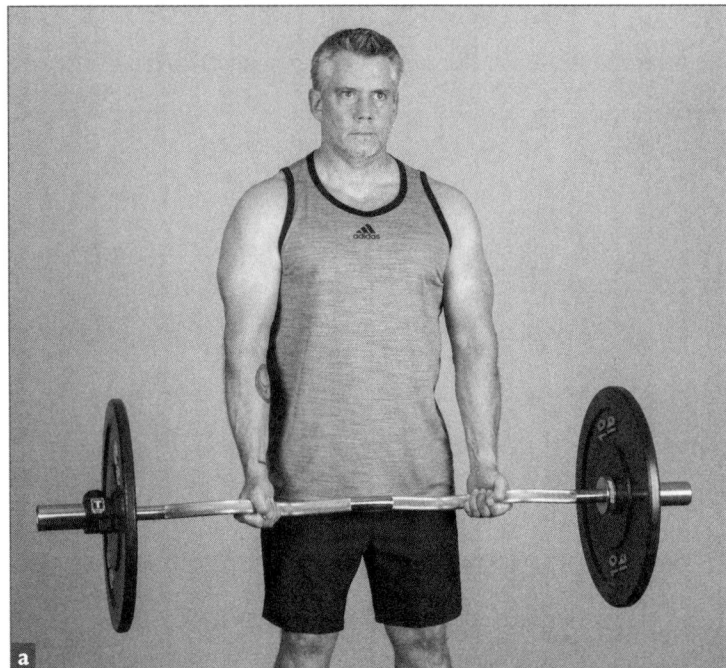

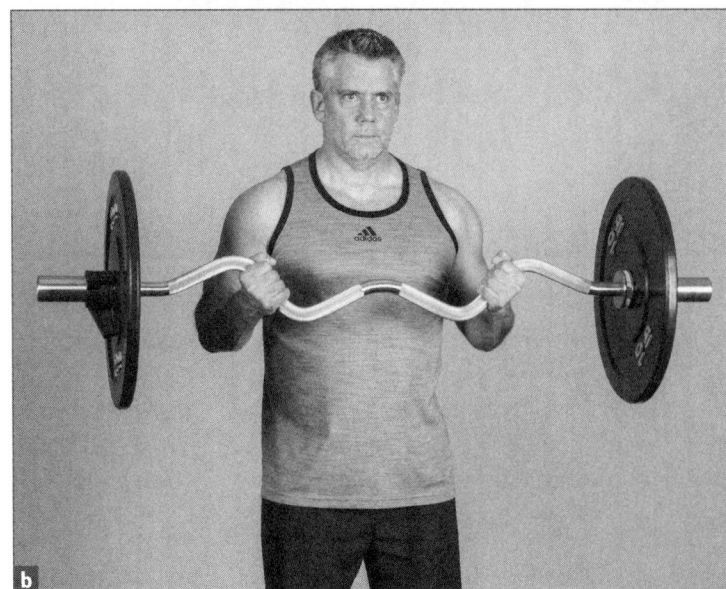

CHAD'S TAKE

Try to keep your elbows at your side or even slightly behind your body as you curl up to chest level to help keep tension on the arms without assistance from the shoulders, which can happen at the top of a curl if the elbows come forward. As with all curling variations, I flex my triceps in the bottom position to both maintain tension on the arm muscles while in the stretch position and to ensure I've done a full range of motion each rep. Also, take care not to rest the bar against your body at the bottom, but instead hold the bar slightly in front of you.

Dumbbell Concentration Curl

The concentration curl aims to eliminate help from other body parts and "concentrate" tension on the biceps. It's similar to a preacher curl, incline curl, and spider curl because of the positioning of the upper arm against the inner thigh. If your gym doesn't have an incline bench or preacher bench, these are a great option for biceps focus!

INSTRUCTION

- Sit on a bench with your legs spread and a dumbbell between your feet.
- Grasp the dumbbell with one hand, palm facing away from your body, and rest your elbow against your inner thigh (figure *a*).
- Curl the dumbbell toward your shoulder, keeping your elbow stationary (figure *b*).
- Slowly lower the dumbbell back to the starting position and repeat. When finished, do the same number of reps with the opposite arm.

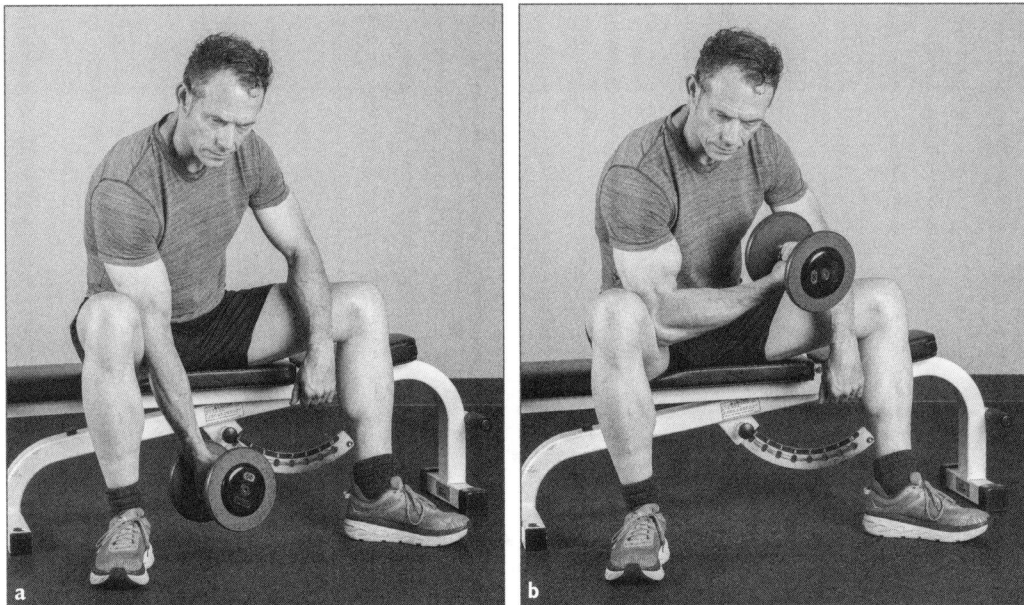

CHAD'S TAKE

An old-school favorite of Arnold Schwarzenegger's, the dumbbell concentration curl is especially good if you have only lighter dumbbells available because the strict positioning will call for less weight. The only negative is since you do only one arm at a time, your workout will take a bit longer.

Cable EZ Curl

The cable curl is a versatile biceps exercise thanks to the nearly endless attachments you can find: single-arm, both arms, ropes, straight, EZ-curl, and more. My favorite is the EZ-bar attachment because it's easier on the wrist than a straight bar.

INSTRUCTION

- Connect an EZ-bar attachment to a low cable pulley.
- Grasp the bar with an underhand, slightly supinated grip (the EZ bar has bends for this position), hands shoulder-width apart (figure a).
- Curl the bar toward your chest, keeping your elbows back and stationary (figure b).
- Slowly lower the bar back to the starting position and repeat.

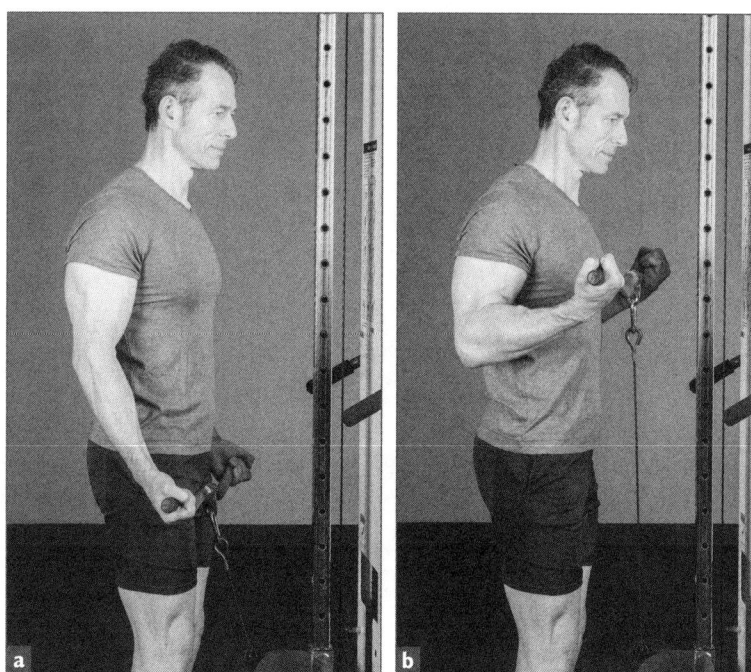

CHAD'S TAKE

I love cables for biceps. The continuous tension throughout the range of motion makes this a staple for me and my clients. I do not like a straight bar on these for the same reason I don't like curling with a straight barbell...many people do not have enough flexibility to turn the palms up enough to find a straight bar comfortable. You can also do these single-armed with a D handle or similar. This is a great option if one arm is considerably stronger than the other. If so, do the weaker arm first and match the weight and reps of the weaker side with the stronger side. Resist the urge to do more on the stronger side. Instead, progress at the pace of the weaker side until it catches up.

Incline Dumbbell Curl

The incline dumbbell curl is a very common biceps exercise; however, I think many people lean the bench back too far. Somewhere between 60 to 75 degrees on the bench will allow the upper arm to hang straight down from the shoulder but slightly behind the body. This will place more tension on the biceps than standing curl variations.

INSTRUCTION

- Sit on an incline bench (approximately 60-degree incline) and hold a dumbbell in each hand, palms facing forward (figure *a*).
- With your arms fully extended and elbows close to your body, curl the dumbbells toward your shoulders (figure *b*).
- Slowly lower the dumbbells back to the starting position and repeat.

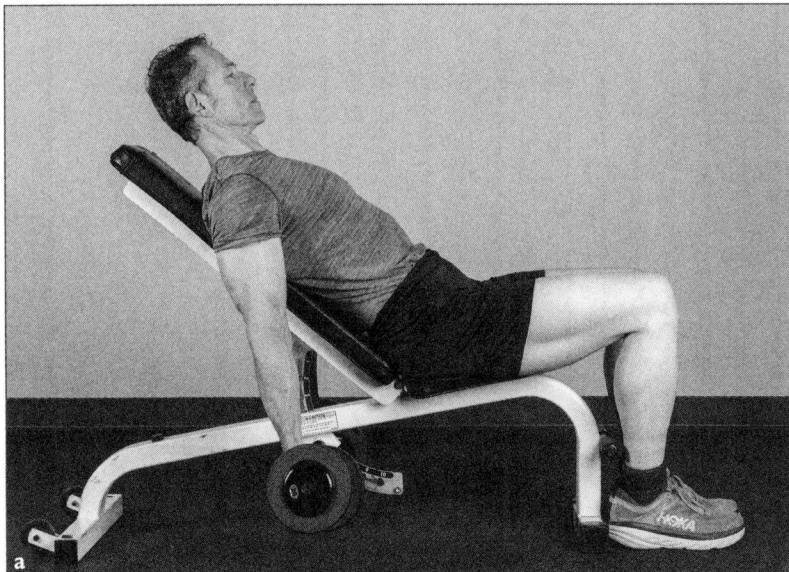

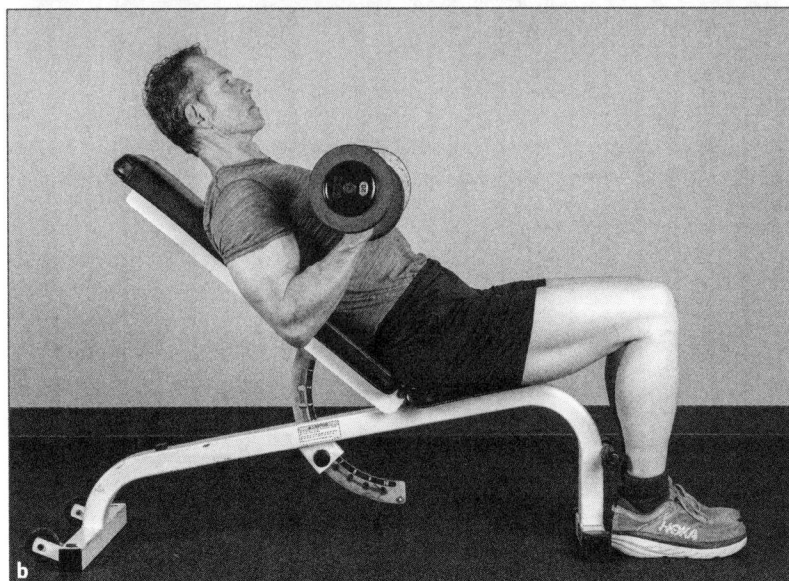

CHAD'S TAKE
You do not need an extreme incline on this exercise; it can put too much stress on the arms and shoulders. If your arms cannot hang straight down perpendicular to the floor, you've reclined the bench too far. This exercise is a good alternative when only lighter weights are available, because the angle of the arm and seated position minimizes the help from other muscles as you curl, thus necessitating lighter weights.

Dumbbell Spider Curl

The dumbbell spider curl is an obscure but effective biceps blaster. It can feel a bit awkward facing down on an incline bench, but the positioning allows for great biceps isolation. If you have trouble connecting to your arm muscles with traditional curling exercises, give this one a try.

INSTRUCTION

- Lie face down on an incline bench at about a 45-degree angle, allowing your arms to hang straight down toward the ground.
- Grasp a pair of dumbbells with an underhand grip, hands shoulder-width apart (figure *a*).
- Curl the weight toward your chest, keeping your elbows stationary and your upper arms perpendicular to the ground (figure *b*).
- Slowly lower the weight back to the starting position and repeat.

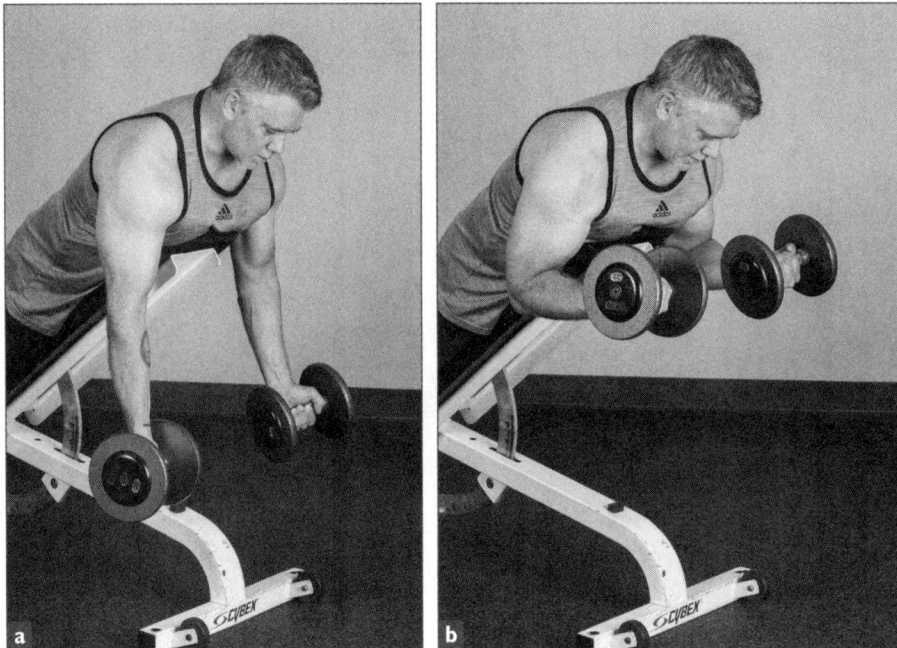

CHAD'S TAKE

The hanging arm position makes it feel similar to a concentration curl or a preacher curl. Because you won't be getting any momentum in this position, you won't be able to go too heavy, which is perfect if you have only lighter dumbbells available at your gym.

TRICEPS EXERCISES

The *triceps brachii* is a three-headed muscle (lateral, medial, and long head) responsible for extending the elbow joint. Strengthening the triceps will improve pushing strength (horizontal like bench press and vertical like overhead pressing) and overall arm aesthetics.

The triceps is one of my favorite muscles to train. First, the triceps takes up about two-thirds of the upper arm, so if you want big arms, well-developed triceps are way more important than biceps. Second, the three heads of the triceps form a horseshoe shape on the back of the arm. For my clients, it's often the first hint of muscle definition they see. Both the men and the women I've trained love seeing that horseshoe. Use the exercises that follow to build your own 'shoes!

Close-Grip Barbell Bench Press

As the name implies, this is a variation of the traditional barbell bench press. With the elbows-in position of the arms, this version minimizes chest-muscle involvement and focuses more on triceps strength. You'll be able to lift much heavier on this exercise than other triceps exercises. If you want big triceps, put this one in the rotation for sure.

INSTRUCTION

- Lie on a flat bench and grasp a barbell with a grip slightly narrower than shoulder-width, palms facing away from you.
- Lower the barbell to your midchest, keeping your elbows close to your body (figure a).
- Press the barbell back up to the starting position (figure b) and repeat.

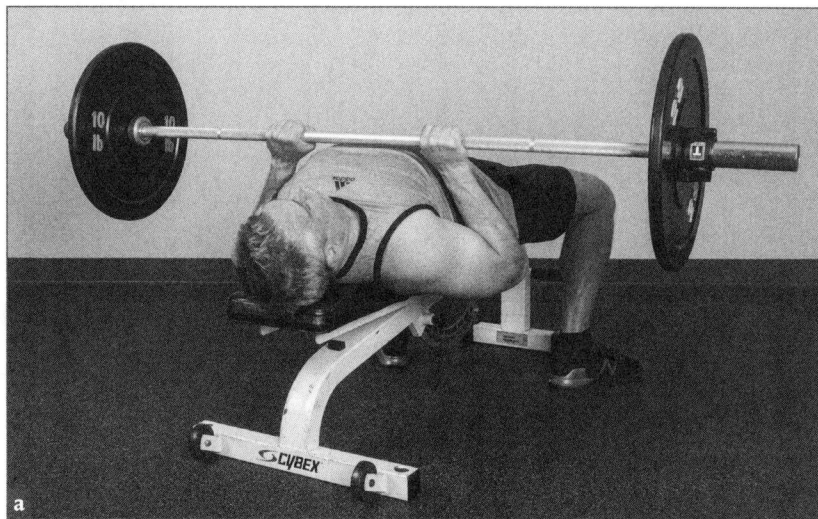

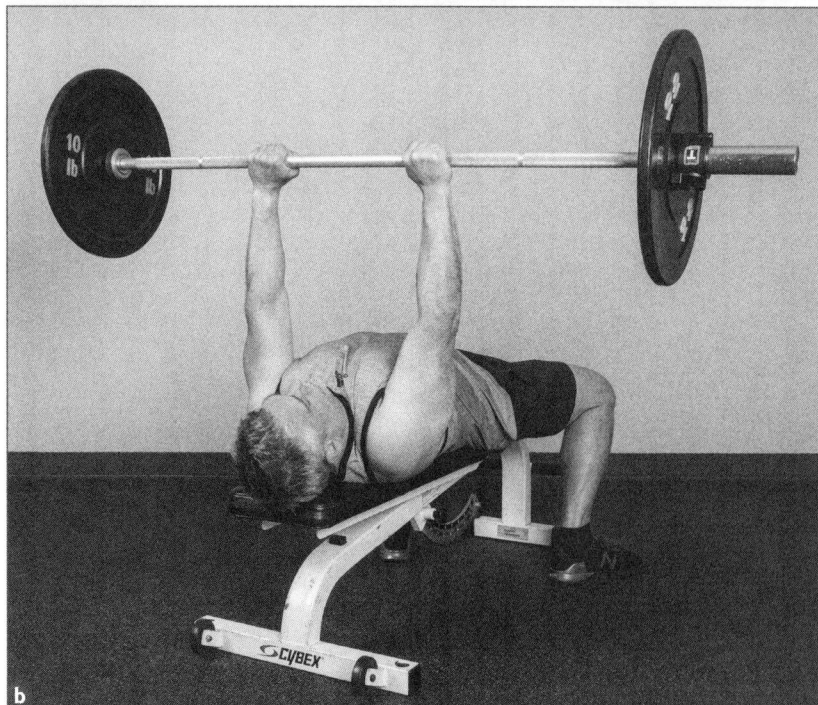

CHAD'S TAKE

I use the close-grip barbell bench press mainly during powerlifting training on my second pressing day of the week. Nonpowerlifters doing full body workouts may want to sub these for a chest press rather than do them on the same day as a chest press later in the workout. The elbow position makes this easier on the shoulders than the regular bench press, so some older trainees may opt for this variation if they want to barbell bench press with a lower risk of shoulder injury.

Triceps Dip

The triceps dip is the granddaddy of triceps exercises and also hits the chest pretty hard. It can be extremely hard to do, especially if you aren't very strong yet or are carrying a lot of body weight. If you have any preexisting shoulder or elbow pain, skip this until you get stronger and your pain subsides.

INSTRUCTION

- Position yourself between parallel bars or V bars with your hands gripping the bars and your legs extended below you. As an alternative, you can bend your knees and hold your feet up behind you, ankles crossed or not (figure *a*).
- Lower your body by bending your elbows until the backs of your upper arms are parallel to the ground if you can. It's OK to stop shy of parallel if you feel pain doing the full range of motion (figure *b*).
- Press through your hands to return to the starting position and repeat.

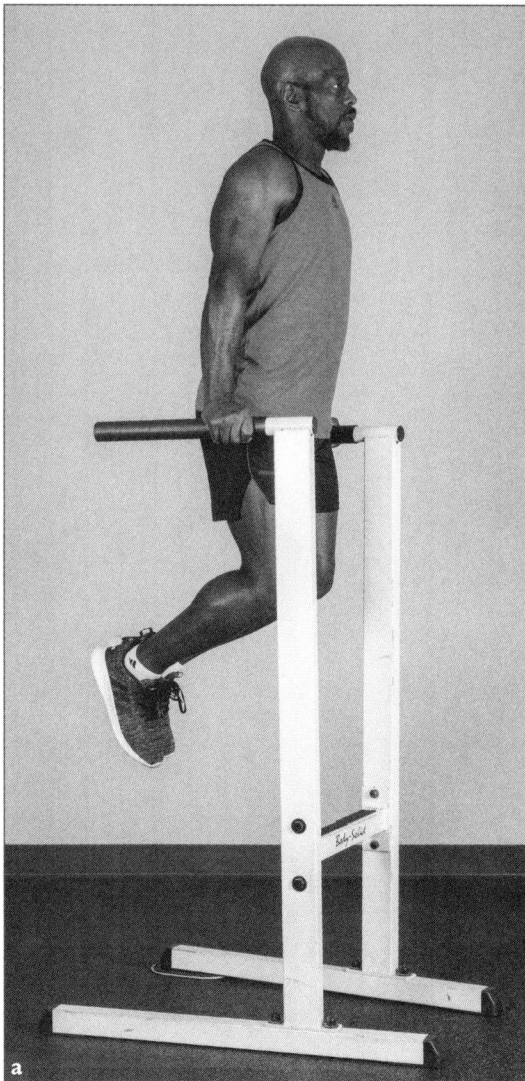

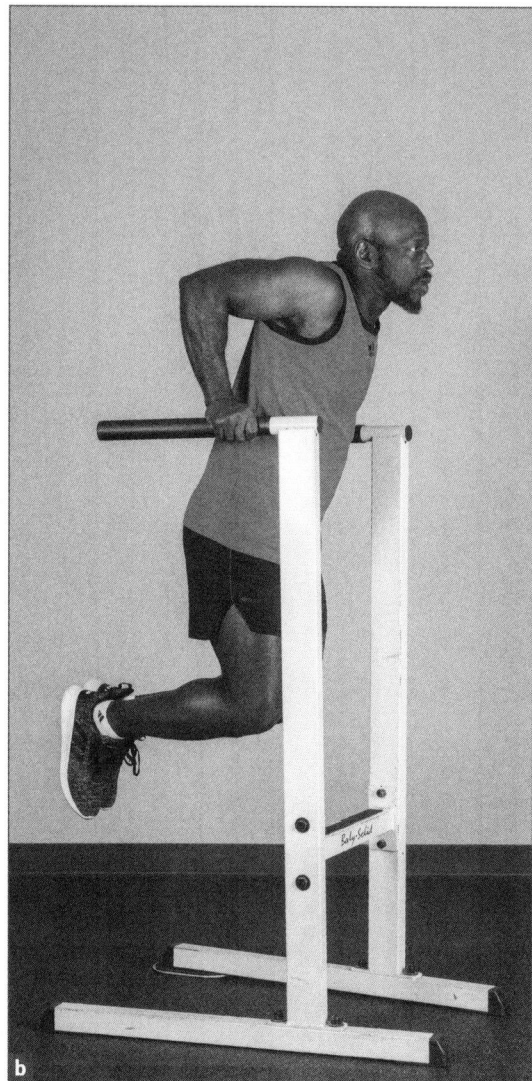

CHAD'S TAKE

Sometimes called the upper-body squat, triceps dips are very hard. You may want to start with other triceps exercises and build up to dips. While I never ban an exercise based on someone's age, older trainees, especially those with preexisting shoulder issues, need to earn the ability to try this exercise. I have an assisted-dip machine that allows clients to counterbalance most of their body weight so they can learn proper form and feel safe when performing dips. If you don't have one of these machines, you can use elastic bands as a counterbalance, but I find them tedious. (Note: I do not like rear bench dips where the arms are behind the body with the hands on a bench behind you, because I find them too strenuous on the shoulder joints.)

Dumbbell Skull Crusher

This is another old-school exercise known by multiple names: skull crusher, nose buster, lying triceps extension. I prefer to use dumbbells for this exercise because there is less chance of actually crushing my skull or busting my nose than when using an EZ-curl bar, but the EZ-curl bar version is fine if you use a spotter or stop well short of failure for safety.

INSTRUCTION

- Lie on a flat bench and grasp a pair of dumbbells with a neutral, palms-in grip, hands shoulder-width apart.
- Extend your arms straight above your chest (figure *a*).
- Bend your elbows, lowering the weight toward your forehead while keeping your upper arms stationary (figure *b*).
- Extend your arms back to the starting position and repeat.

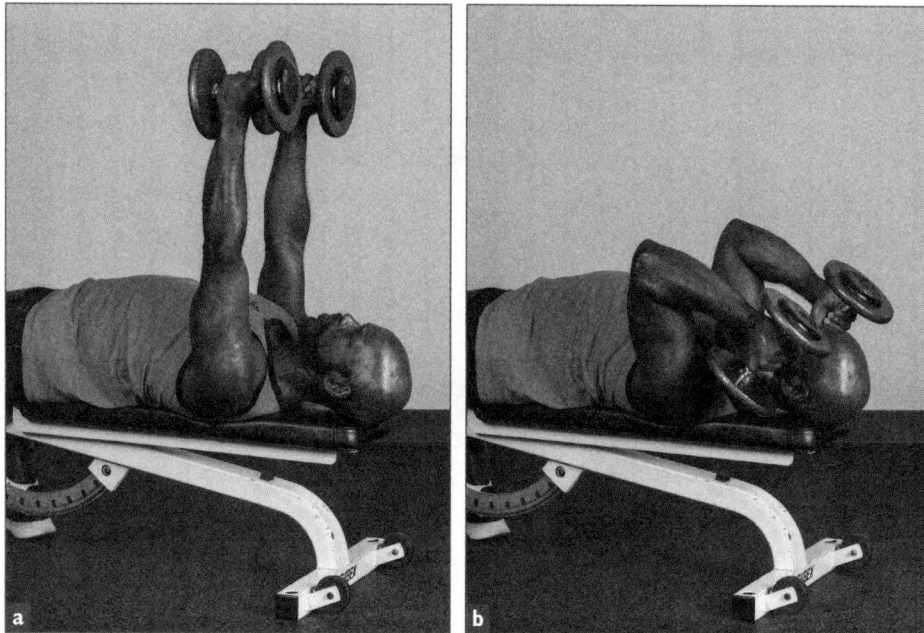

CHAD'S TAKE

I like to bring the weights down past the top of my head rather than to my forehead or nose as in the more traditional exercise to get more range of motion. I do this by allowing my upper arm to go back almost parallel to the floor in the stretch position instead of keeping the upper arm relatively stable and perpendicular to the floor as in a strict skullcrusher. I also like to keep the upper arm angled slightly less than vertical at the top of the movement to keep more tension on the triceps and prevent taking a bit of rest each rep at the top.

Cable Triceps Push-Down

This is my favorite triceps exercise using a cable stack. It hits all three heads of the triceps well, is easy to learn, and provides a surprising stimulus on the core as the weights get heavier. I prefer to keep my elbows back at the top of the movement, but many people let their hands and elbows come too high at the top of the exercise and "fling" the weight down with assistance from the lats. Don't do this—keep your form strict and focus on the triceps.

INSTRUCTION

- Attach a straight bar or rope to a high cable pulley.
- Grasp the attachment with an overhand grip, hands shoulder-width apart at chest level (figure *a*).
- With your elbows close to your body, push the attachment downward until your arms are fully extended (figure *b*).
- Slowly return to the starting position at chest level and repeat.

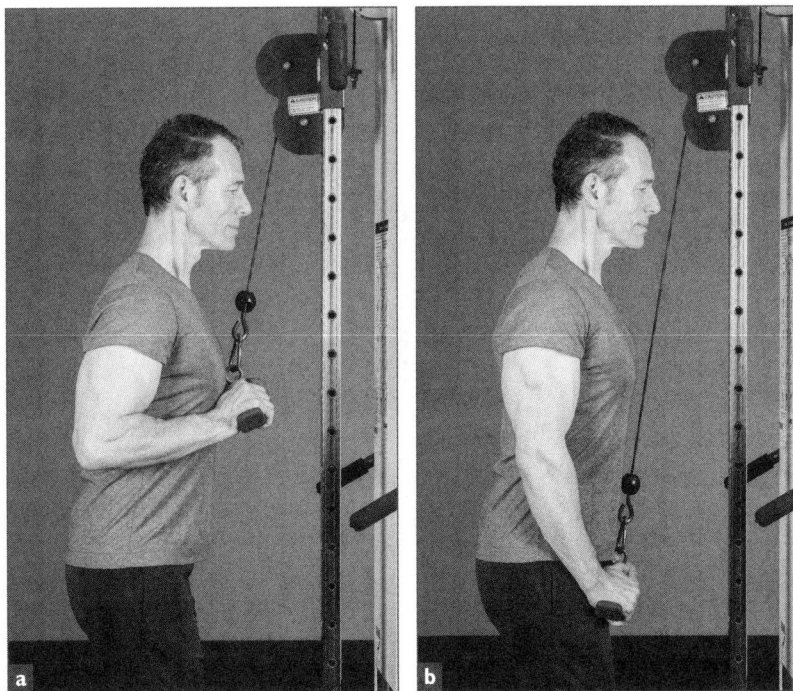

CHAD'S TAKE

I love this exercise! I prefer a slightly angled bar if available because it's more comfortable on the wrists than a straight bar. Also, fatter handles are more comfortable on the hands if you have one available. The rope option is great too, but note you'll probably need to use lighter weight due to leverage differences. Also, I like single-arm versions of this one, which can be done with a pronated, supinated, or neutral grip depending on what attachments you have available and what feels best on your joints. All three grips do the same thing, so there is no need to do multiple sets with each one.

Elbows-In Push-Up

A great push-up variation for those desiring more triceps work, especially if you have a limited gym and rely on body-weight exercises.

INSTRUCTION

- Get into a push-up position with your hands close together and elbows at your sides (figure *a*). (Those who lack wrist flexibility may prefer to use push-up handles to help keep the wrists in a more neutral position.)
- Lower your body by bending your elbows until your chest is close to the ground (figure *b*).
- Press through your hands to return to the starting position and repeat.

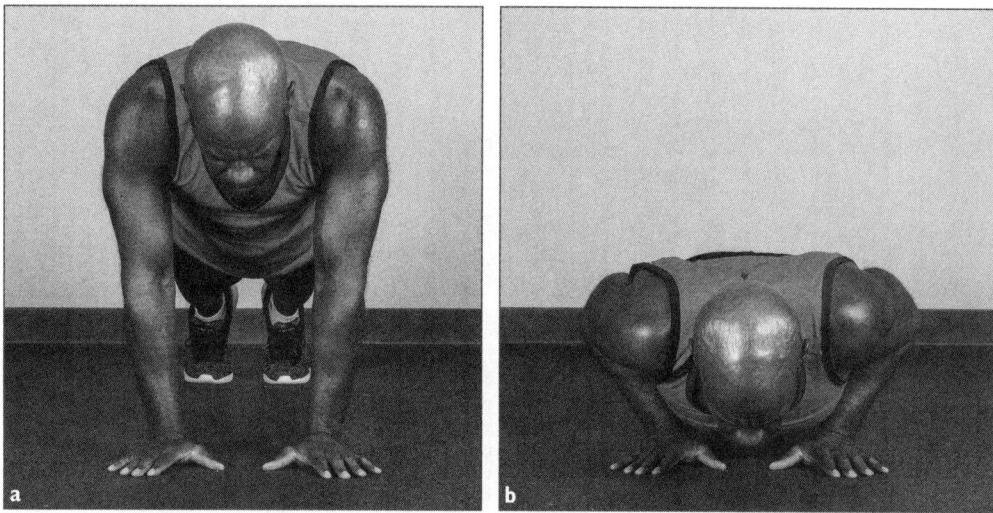

CHAD'S TAKE

For those who have the strength to do it, this exercise is a great triceps developer. The elbows-in push-up is a more difficult exercise than a traditional push-up because of less pec involvement, so it may be best to start with other exercises and build up to this one. You may want to start these on a bar in a rack to lessen the body weight you'll need to lift.

Single-Arm Dumbbell Kickback

Perhaps the most widely seen arm exercise in pop culture, nearly every film, TV show, or commercial set in a gym will invariably depict someone doing a triceps kickback with a two-pound weight. The leverage on this exercise doesn't typically allow for very heavy weights, so you'll probably outgrow the usefulness of this exercise fairly quickly.

INSTRUCTION

- Hold a dumbbell in one hand and place the opposite hand and knee on a bench.
- Bend at the waist, keeping your back straight, and lift the weighted arm parallel to the ground with a 90-degree bend in the elbow (figure *a*).
- Extend your arm back, straightening your elbow, while keeping your upper arm stationary (figure *b*).
- Slowly return to the starting position and repeat. Switch arms after completing the desired number of reps.

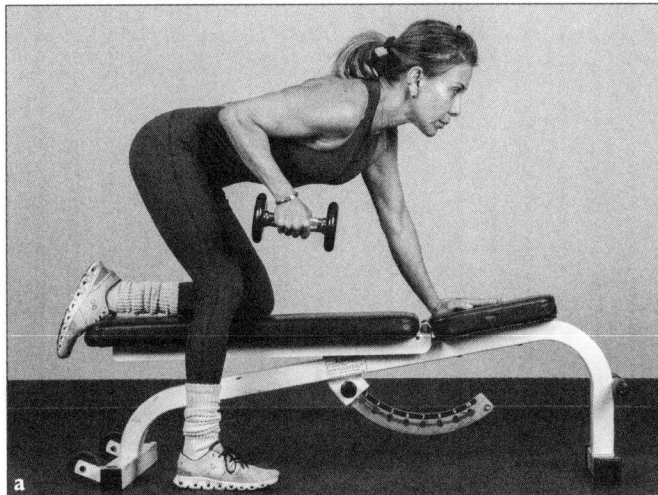

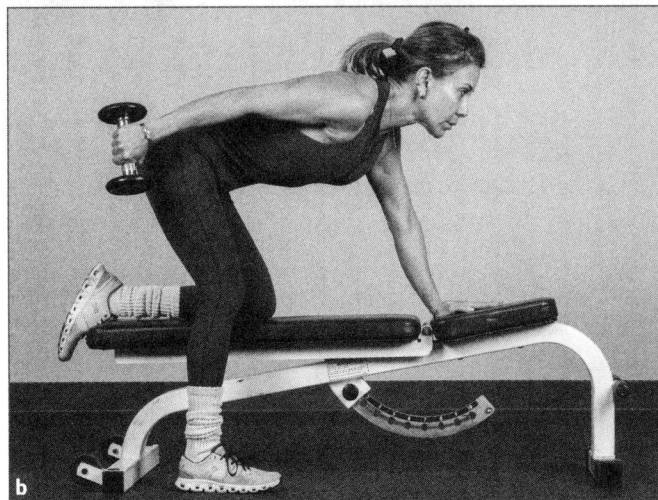

CHAD'S TAKE

I prefer other triceps exercises, but if I were to do the single-arm kickback, I'd likely use cables instead of dumbbells. That being said, those with limited equipment and access to only lighter dumbbells may find this exercise to be a great alternative.

Cable Overhead Triceps Extension

Overhead extensions are great for overall triceps development, but the position can be difficult for those who lack shoulder flexion. Also, some people's shoulder or elbow joints protest a bit in the overhead position, so as great of a muscle builder as this is, don't use it if it's not comfortable on your joints.

INSTRUCTION

- Attach a rope or bar to a low cable pulley.
- Grasp the attachment with both hands, palms facing each other or down, face away from the machine and step forward to create tension in the cable (figure *a*).
- With your elbows close to your ears, extend your arms above your head, straightening your elbows (figure *b*).
- Slowly return to the starting position and repeat.

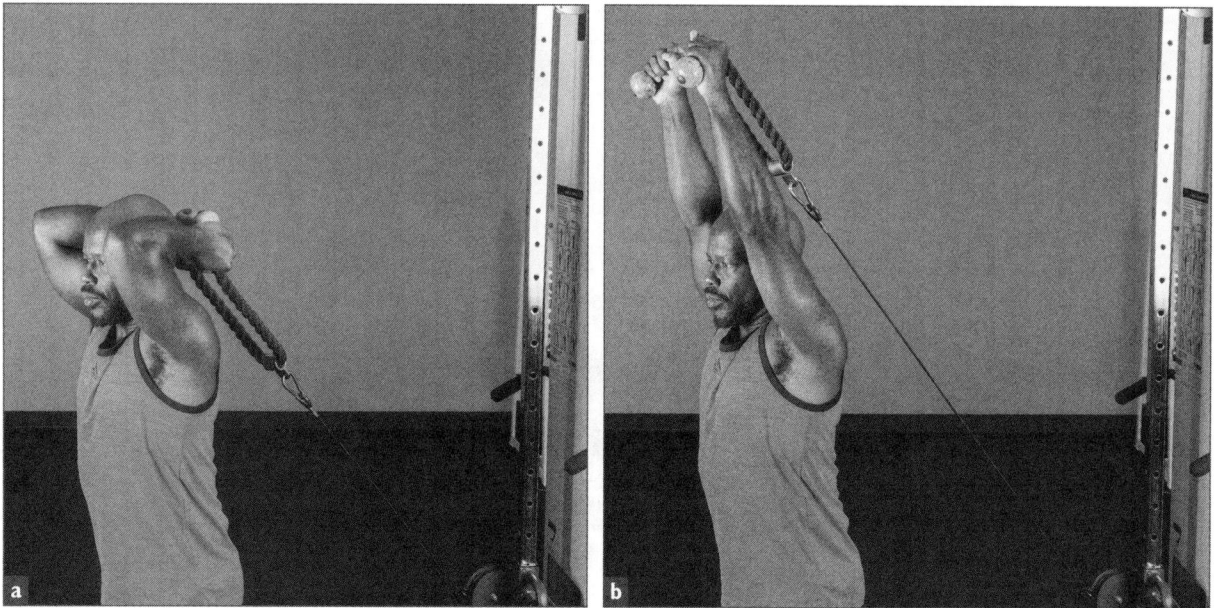

CHAD'S TAKE

If comfortable on your shoulders, overhead triceps movements are a great stimulant of triceps development. I like single-arm versions of this exercise as well. You can do these with a dumbbell if a cable system is unavailable, but I prefer the continuous tension throughout the range of motion that cables provide.

Dumbbell Tate Press

The Tate press is named after famed powerlifter Dave Tate. It's an exercise common to powerlifting gyms and programs because the heavy triceps work it provides makes it a great assistance exercise for the bench press.

INSTRUCTION

- Lie on a flat bench and hold a pair of dumbbells above your chest with your palms facing your feet (figure *a*).
- Bend your elbows and lower the dumbbells toward your chest, keeping the dumbbells touching throughout the movement (figure *b*).
- Press the dumbbells back to the starting position and repeat.

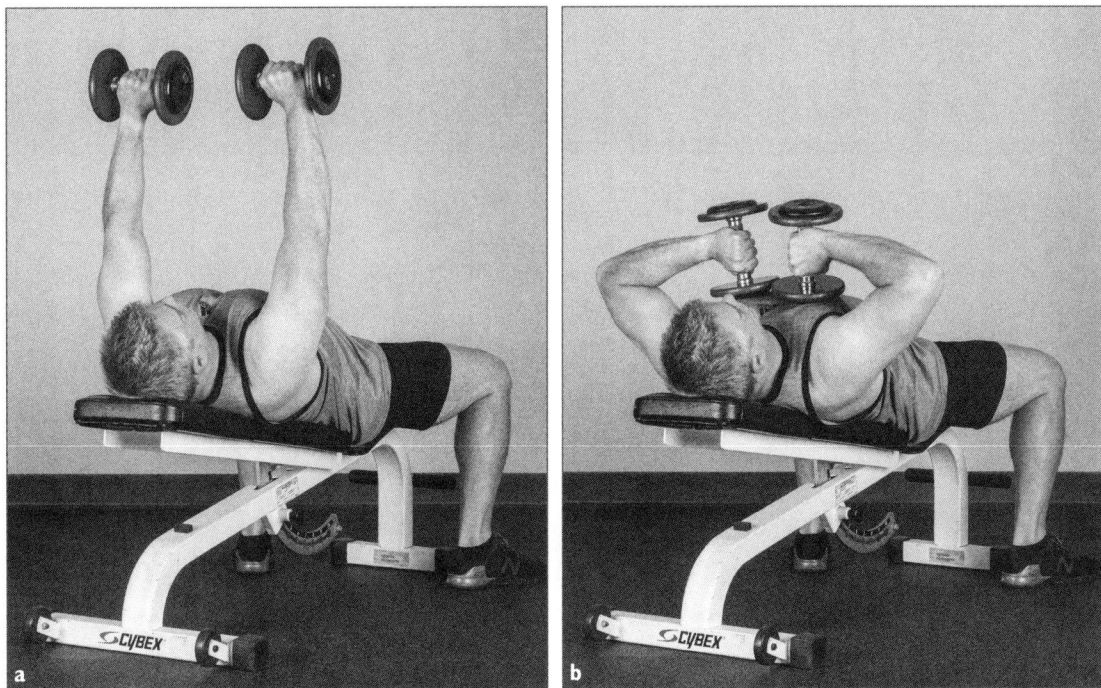

CHAD'S TAKE

I prefer doing these on a 30- to 45-degree incline bench but do what feels most comfortable to you. There's no real benefit to the angle other than comfort, but for those of us over 50, comfort can determine whether we use an exercise or not. Do what feels best for you!

CHAPTER 8

Core

Six-pack abs. That's the first image that comes to mind when most people think about their core. And while there's nothing wrong with aspiring to have Brad Pitt's *Fight Club* midsection, the core is so much more than a great six-pack.

Although attaining a visible six-pack can be motivating, it's accomplished more by dieting off the body fat covering the abdominal muscles than by doing any particular ab exercise or routine. And if we're honest, most of us over age 50 don't really care if we ever have a six-pack, but we do care that we are strong enough to enjoy our leisure time—gardening, playing with kids or grandkids, taking adventure vacations—without injuring our backs. So while it doesn't matter if you never get lean enough for a six-pack, the muscles of the core are one of the most important areas to focus on when it comes to overall strength and stability. A strong core supports good posture, protects the spine, and improves overall athletic performance.

Traditionally, core work consisted of endless sit-ups or crunch variations (some folks call them curl-ups). And while those exercises do work the six-pack muscle, called the *rectus abdominis*, there are other muscles just as important for strength and stability of the torso. Think of the core like a three-dimensional cylinder, with the rectus abdominis on the front, the obliques on the sides, the muscles of the lower back in rear, and even a top (the diaphragm) and bottom (the pelvic floor). Endless crunches are simply not going to work all those muscles.

I do very little crunching with clients or in my own training. The bulk of the work we do is about *preventing* motion, not causing it. We focus more on bracing the core and not allowing the spine to move front to back (sagittal plane), side to side (frontal plane), or rotationally (transverse plane). Bracing is simply "bearing down" as you might do if you were going to allow your kid to punch you in the gut. You don't want to suck in your stomach or hold your breath—just brace.

My best abdominal development occurred in my 40s when I began powerlifting. My core musculature got an intense stimulus from bracing on all the heavy sets of squats, bench presses, and deadlifts I did. In fact, for a decade I did almost no direct abdominal work, yet I could still demonstrate even the most difficult core exercise to a new client.

However, most of you reading this book likely have no desire to be a powerlifter or employ the heavy weights I was lifting (300-pound squat, 300-pound bench, and 400-pound deadlift). For you, I recommend the exercises and programs that follow. You certainly don't need to have a devoted ab day, but you do want to make sure your core is 3D strong!

I'm not in the camp that says you can never flex the spine, and I have no problem with having some spinal flexion (and extension for that matter) in a program. But I don't feel that flexion needs to be a very big part of your routine, and certainly not a focus, like doing hundreds of crunches a day.

The following 11 exercises are great for building a strong core. Myriad others exist, but master these before trying something crazy you saw on YouTube! And yes, I even included a couple crunch variations because I know many of you will want to do them no matter what I say.

Stir the Pot

This is my favorite core exercise (and the favorite of renowned spinal researcher Dr. Stuart McGill, from whom I learned it). You'll need a Swiss ball (aka stability ball) for this one. It stimulates bracing of the core in all three planes: sagittal, transverse, and frontal. For this reason, if I could only do one core exercise, this would be it!

INSTRUCTION

- Start in a plank position with your forearms resting on an exercise ball. Most people do best with a 55- or 65-centimeter ball.
- Move the ball in a circular motion, alternating 10 to 15 reps done clockwise followed by the same number of reps done counterclockwise.

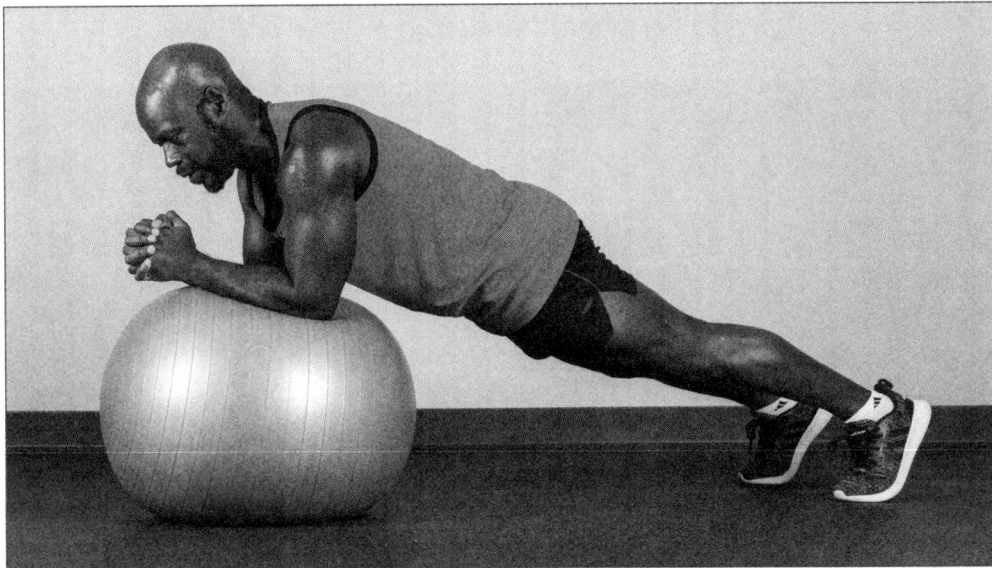

CHAD'S TAKE

Start with your feet as wide as you need to to feel stable and safe and learn the exercise. As you get stronger, try narrowing your feet; this will make you less stable and thus make the exercise harder. Another option I call "push the pot" is to simply move the elbows forward and backward instead of in a circular motion. It's nearly as difficult with less fear of losing your balance. If you get really strong, try putting your feet on a balance pad on either version to really up the intensity!

Pallof Press

This favorite is specifically for "anti-rotation." In it we are bracing the core to prevent rotation of the spine in the transverse plane. This works the oblique muscles on the sides very effectively.

INSTRUCTION

- Stand perpendicular to a cable machine with the cable at chest height using a single-arm attachment.
- Hold onto the handle with both hands (I prefer to interlace my fingers, but some prefer to overlap hands) and extend arms straight out in front so there is a 90-degree angle between the cable and your outstretched arms (figure a).
- Slowly pull the cable back toward the chest (figure b), engaging the core throughout for 10 to 15 reps on each side.

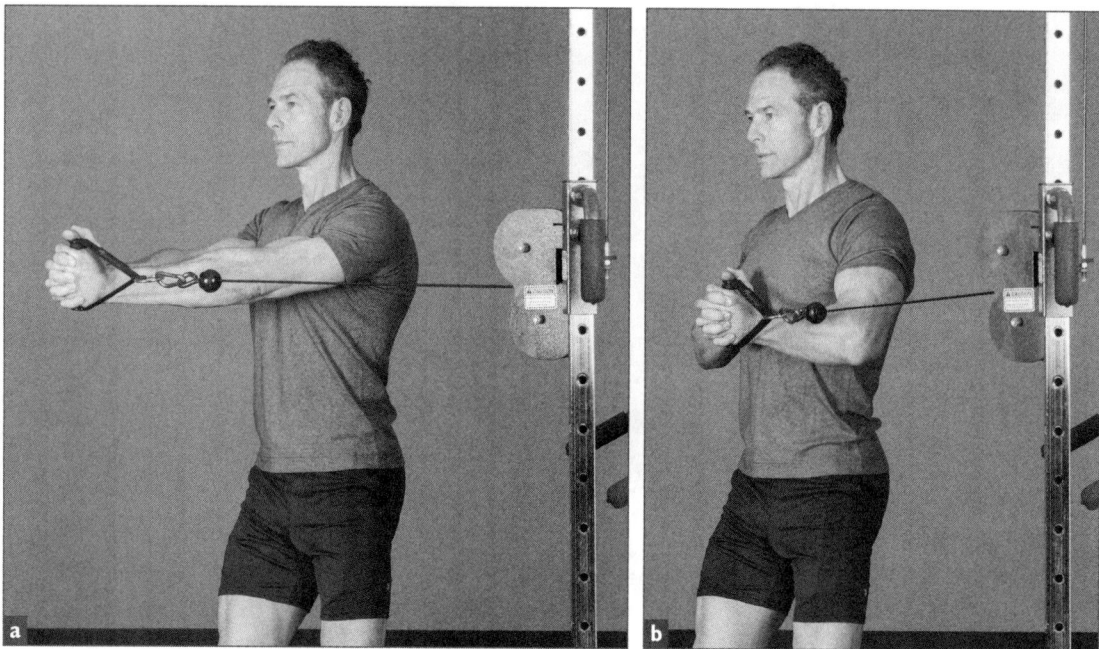

CHAD'S TAKE

The Pallof press is my top exercise for anti-rotation, but I like the "hold" version even better! The hold version is done for time in the arms-outstretched position of the Pallof press and is much more difficult than the press. Aim for at least 30 seconds on each side before trying a heavier weight. Think about bracing the core and feeling the obliques preventing your spine from rotating. Start on the side opposite your baseball or softball batting stance because it will likely be the weaker side. Simply match the reps of the weaker side with the stronger side. Stop even if you could do more with the stronger side and allow the weaker side to catch up. I've found this exercise helpful for older clients because most have never thought about core strength in the transverse plane. The ability to control your spine when it rotates, or to prevent rotating at all, is important as we age and might spend more time traveling or gardening, situations where we could be carrying unsteady loads on uneven or slippery surfaces.

Farmer Walk

The farmer walk is our most basic exercise to prevent lateral flexion (bending to the side) of our spine. You must brace your core in this exercise, so it is quite applicable to the real world, especially if you want to carry *all* the grocery bags in one trip!

The farmer walk is somewhat easy because the loads you carry are balanced. As such, you'll be able to carry more weight than on the more difficult suitcase carry (which I also recommend). As the name implies, the load is carried on one side only, like carrying a suitcase—at least in the days before everything had wheels. The side of the abdomen opposite the load will need to work harder to prevent your spine from bending laterally toward the load side.

INSTRUCTION

- Pick up a heavy pair of dumbbells or kettlebells, one weight in each hand.
- Walk forward for a set distance or time while keeping core engaged and posture upright. Try going for 30 to 60 meters, yards, or seconds for 2 or 3 rounds.

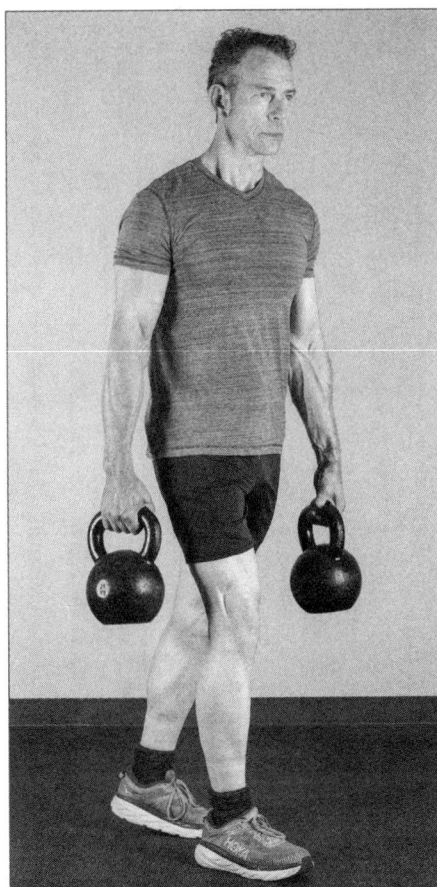

CHAD'S TAKE

The farmer walk will likely be as taxing on your grip strength as it is on your core. But remember, a strong grip is linked to longevity, so don't skip this if your grip is weak when you start out. Progress at the pace your grip strength allows, even if it doesn't feel as taxing on the core. Take care not to shrug the shoulders or bend the elbows excessively. Another option is the suitcase carry. Use the same technique as the farmer walk, but carry a weight in only one hand. Even though you'll only be using half the weight of the farmer walk, the asymmetrical load will light up the muscles on the side of the abdomen opposite the weight.

Dead Bug

This is the first core exercise I teach new clients. While it's technically the easiest antiflexion core exercise, it's often much harder than it appears. There are a few versions floating around the internet. This technique is my favorite.

INSTRUCTION

- Lie on your back on an exercise mat with one arm extended overhead and one arm at your side. Then bring both knees to the chest, bent at about 90 degrees, feet elevated. Then lower the leg on the same side as the "down" arm so it is straight but still off the floor. Think left arm overhead and left knee at the chest, right arm down and right leg out straight. Now you're in the starting position (figure a).

- Slowly switch sides so the arms and legs on each side of the body are now in the opposite position (figure b). Reverse direction and return to the original starting position. Repeat for 10 to 15 reps on each side, engaging the core throughout the motion and keeping the lower back pressed against the mat.

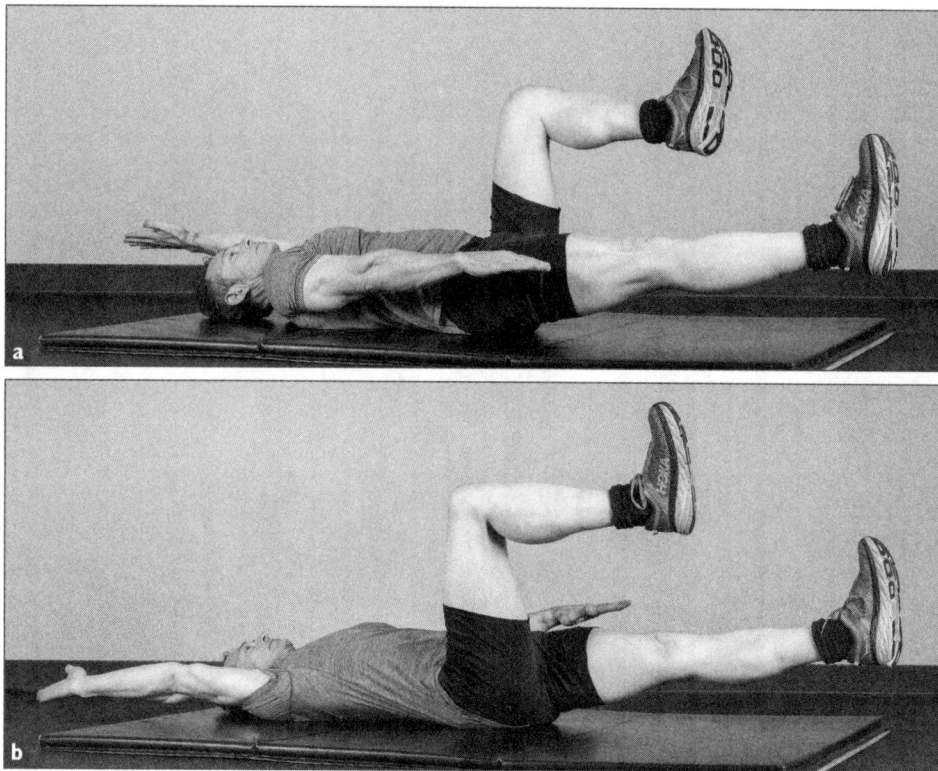

CHAD'S TAKE

There are easier versions of dead bug if this one proves too difficult. Instead of using the same side of the body, use the diagonal opposite: right arm and left knee up with left arm and right leg down. Using opposite sides can be easier to control than using the same side. Another option is to keep the knees bent as you lower them to lightly tap the floor. The bent-knee position shortens the lever considerably over the straight leg. This can make it easier to keep your lower back against the mat during the movement. No matter what option you choose, keep the core braced and the lower back pushed into the mat. It's all about spinal stabilization while the arms and legs move, much like what happens naturally during everyday activities and sports.

Bird Dog

We often forget that the core is a cylinder, and the back side needs to be worked as well. If you're already doing heavy squats and deadlifts, you can probably skip these. I tend to use this exercise more with beginners, geriatric clients, and those recovering from a lower back injury.

INSTRUCTION

- Start on your hands and knees with your back straight and core engaged.
- Extend one arm and extend the opposite leg off the ground, reaching for the walls so the arms, legs, and back are one straight line (figure *a*). Hold for a second or two before lowering back down.
- Do 10 to 15 reps, then repeat on the opposite side (figure *b*).

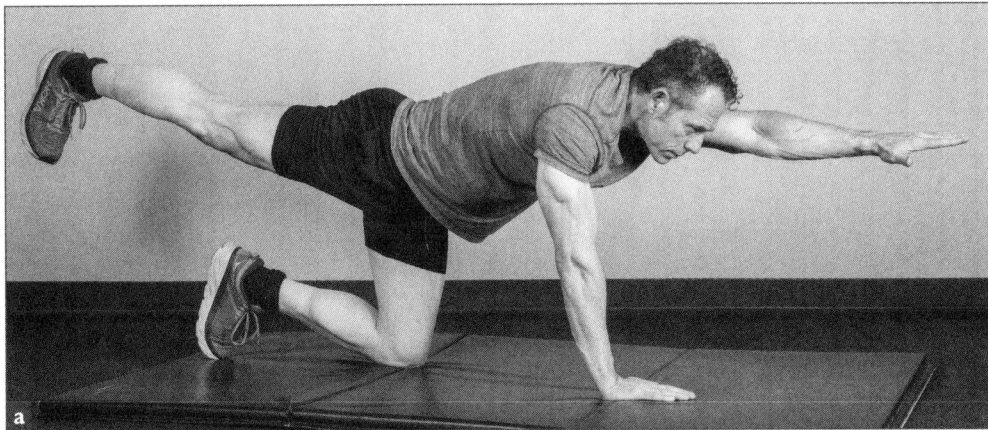

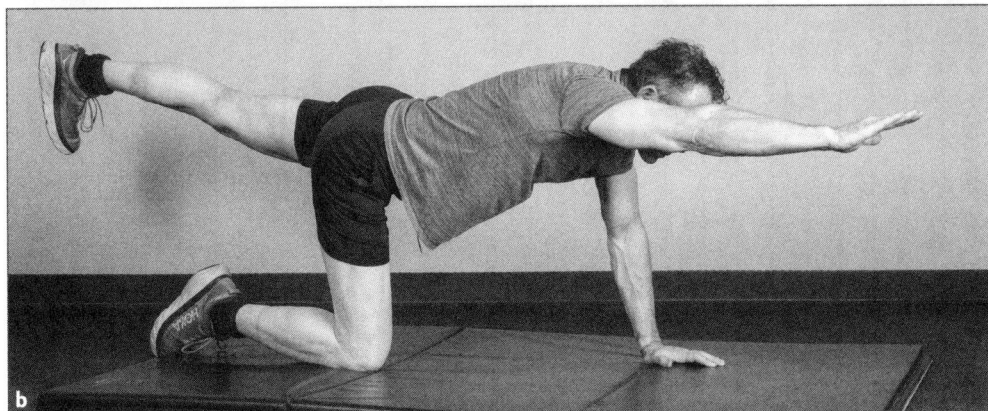

CHAD'S TAKE

Think slow and controlled movements during the bird dog. Endeavor to keep the back flat and reach for the walls with your arms and legs. Many people incorrectly kick their leg up toward the ceiling when doing this exercise, causing the lower back to hyperextend. Don't do that.

Superman

Superman is basically a lying-down version of the bird dog. It doesn't require the same balance or coordination and should be the first option for those with a weak lower back or recovering from injury.

INSTRUCTION

- Lie face down on a mat in a flying position.
- Lift one arm and the opposite leg off the ground (figure *a*) and hold for a second or two.
- Lower to the ground.
- Perform 10 to 15 repetitions on one side and switch sides (figure *b*). If that's too hard, alternating sides should be a bit easier.

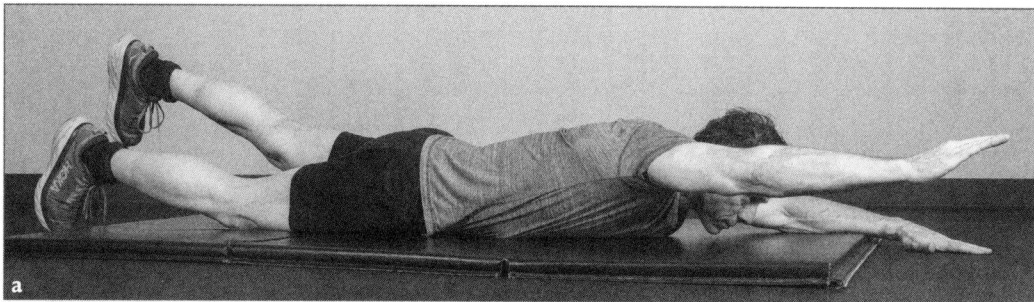

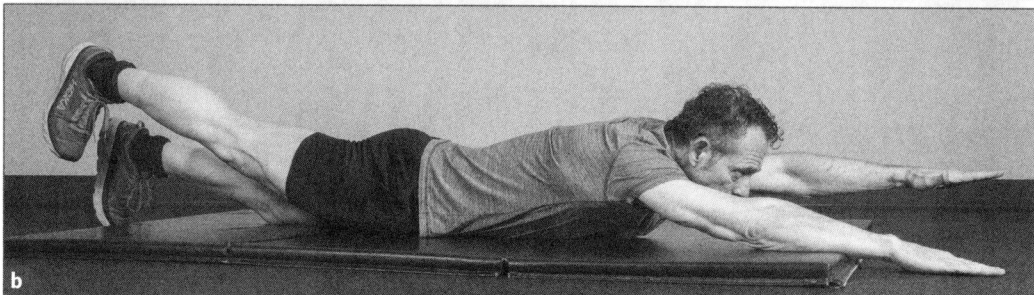

CHAD'S TAKE

Even though this exercise is a bit easier to do than the bird dog, some older trainees who lack shoulder mobility or neck flexibility might not find the position comfortable. A work-around is to try the exercise while lying on a massage table or wide padded weight bench where you might be able to find a more comfortable position for the neck and arms by lying slightly off the front of the bench.

Plank

One of the most recognizable abdominal exercises, the plank is more of a transition exercise, bridging the gap between the easier exercises like dead bug and harder ones like the body saw and stir the pot.

INSTRUCTION

- Start in a push-up position with the elbows or forearms resting on the ground, mat, or Airex pad.
- Keep the back straight and core engaged as you hold the position for up to one minute for 1 to 3 rounds.

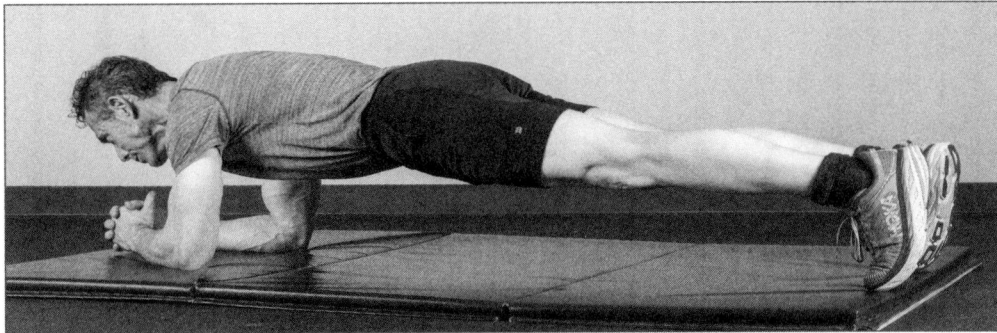

CHAD'S TAKE

Use bracing similar to dead bug. However, this bracing in the plank position is much harder. Master dead bug first and then progress to the plank. Note: Despite the Guinness World Record plank being over nine and a half *hours*, I do not like going longer than 60 seconds on a plank. I think it's a waste of energy, more geared toward endurance than strength. I will either add an external load with a weighted vest (again, only up to 60 seconds), or I'll progress to a harder exercise like stir the pot or body saw.

Body Saw

The body saw is one of my favorites. It ramps up the difficulty of a traditional plank considerably. You will need sliders for these. If you don't have sliders, you can do a similar move to the "push the pot" I mentioned in Chad's Take under stir the pot (page 119).

INSTRUCTION

- Start in a plank position with the feet on exercise sliders and the elbows and forearms resting on the ground, an exercise mat, or an Airex pad. A mat or Airex pad will be much more comfortable than the ground.
- Push back as far as you can with your upper body without allowing the hips to drop (figure *a*), then pull forward to the starting position (figure *b*).
- Repeat for 10 to 15 reps.

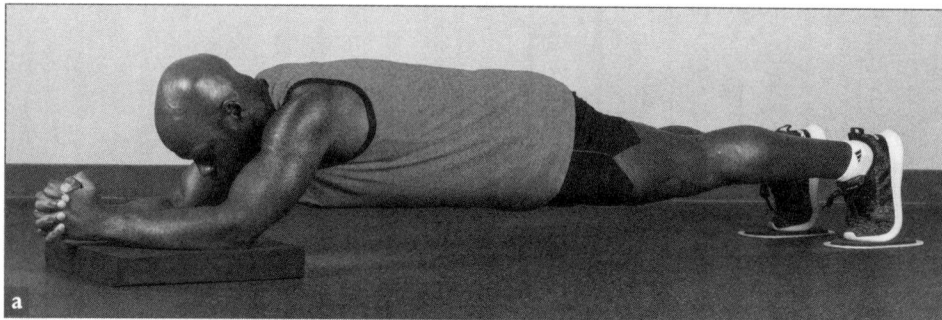

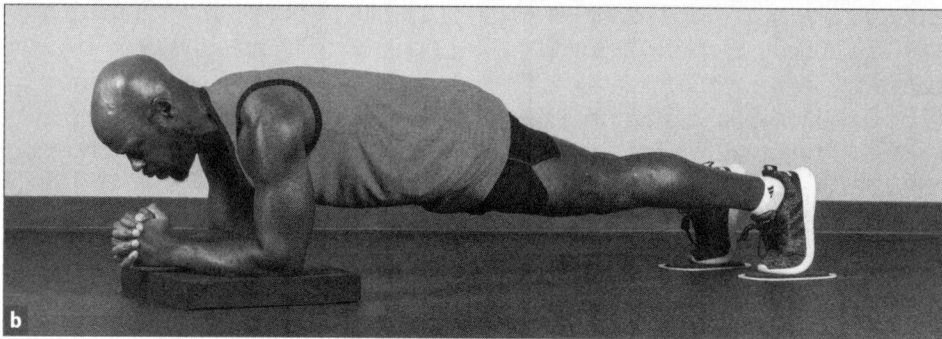

CHAD'S TAKE

The body saw is a much better way to progress a traditional plank than by adding more time. If your gym doesn't have sliders, it's worth it to buy your own so you can try this killer exercise. With stronger clients, I may add a bit of external load via a weight vest.

McGill Crunch

This is the only crunch that spine researcher Dr. Stuart McGill recommends. If I do a crunch, I do the McGill crunch. McGill likes it because the pelvis is stable and the amount of flexion of the spine is minimized compared to the traditional crunch. If a regular crunch doesn't agree with your lower back, this one might allow you to crunch pain-free.

INSTRUCTION

- Lie on your back with one knee bent and that foot flat on the ground and the other leg straight.
- Place your hands underneath your lower back to provide support (figure a).
- Slowly lift your head and shoulders off the ground while keeping the lower back in contact with the hands (figure b).
- Repeat for 10 to 15 reps then switch leg positions and repeat.

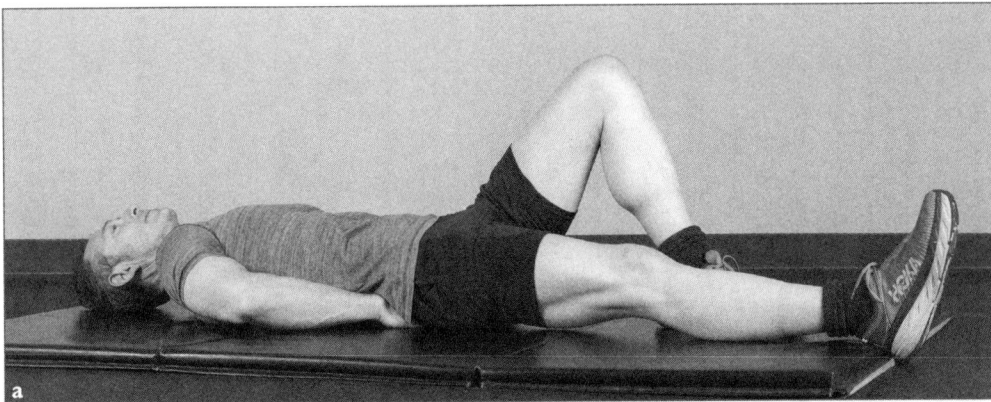

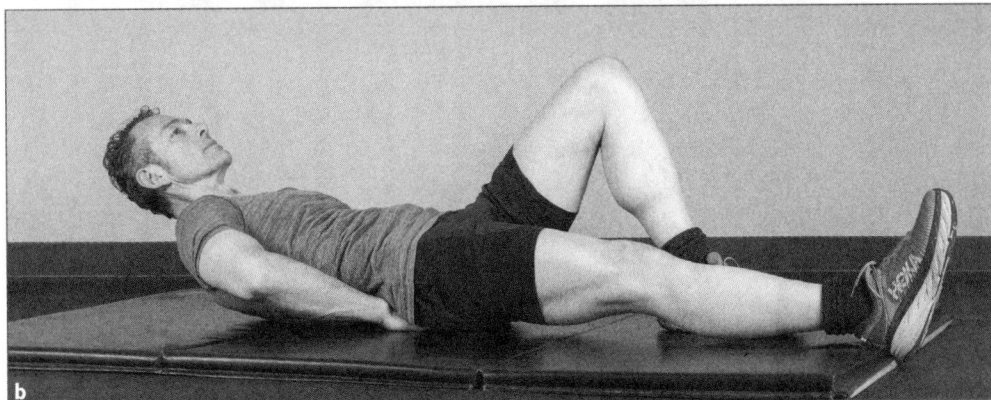

CHAD'S TAKE

This exercise has very short range of motion, and you won't feel like you are doing much until the burn sets in. I recommend very shallow breathing with this. While you don't want to hold your breath, you can't really take in a full breath either. I do little puffs out on the way up, and a short inhale on the way down.

Swiss Ball Crunch

As the name says, you'll need a Swiss ball for this one. Most people will do well with a 55- or 65-centimeter ball. I like this crunch because the curved surface of the ball allows a more thorough range of motion for the rectus abdominis (six-pack muscle) than when crunching on a flat surface.

INSTRUCTION

- Lie back on a Swiss ball with the feet flat on the ground and knees bent. The rear of the pelvis should rest on the top front of the ball and the upper back on the top rear surface.
- Cross the arms over the chest and engage the core muscles (figure *a*).
- Use the abdominal muscles to curl the chest forward toward the hips (figure *b*).
- Repeat for 10 to 15 reps or more.

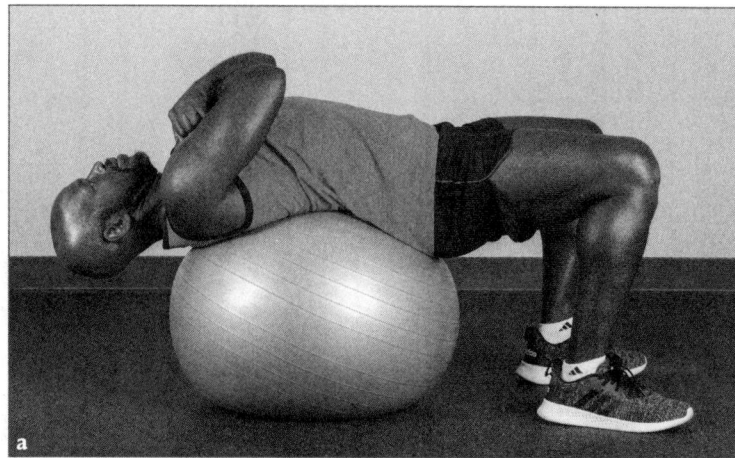

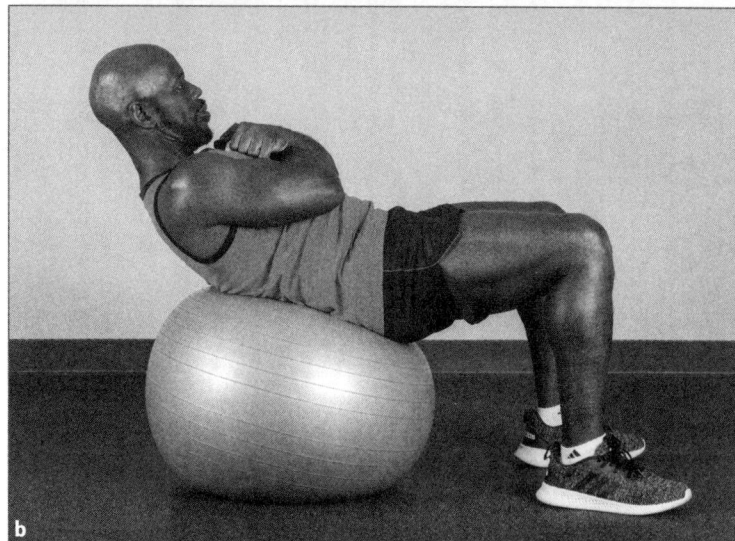

CHAD'S TAKE

Make sure the ball is firm and supports the lower back. You do not want to sit up straight but rather curl yourself over the top of the ball. Bonus points if you can tilt your pelvis toward your chest as you do this. This will essentially pull from both ends of the muscle and maximize the contraction on each rep. A cue I use is to try to look into your belly button, which will get your chest and belly button as close together as possible.

Reverse Crunch

Instead of trying to curl our chest down to our pelvis as in the regular crunch, with the reverse crunch we are trying to curl the pelvis up to the chest. This is much harder, mainly because we carry more weight in the lower body, so it's naturally harder to lift. It's a great exercise to progress to once you've built up a bit of abdominal strength.

INSTRUCTION

- Lie on your back on a flat bench with the hands holding the bench about head level, elbows pointing up (figure a).
- Use the abdominal muscles to lift the hips off the bench, curling the knees toward the chest (figure b).
- Lower to the starting position and repeat for 10 to 15 reps.

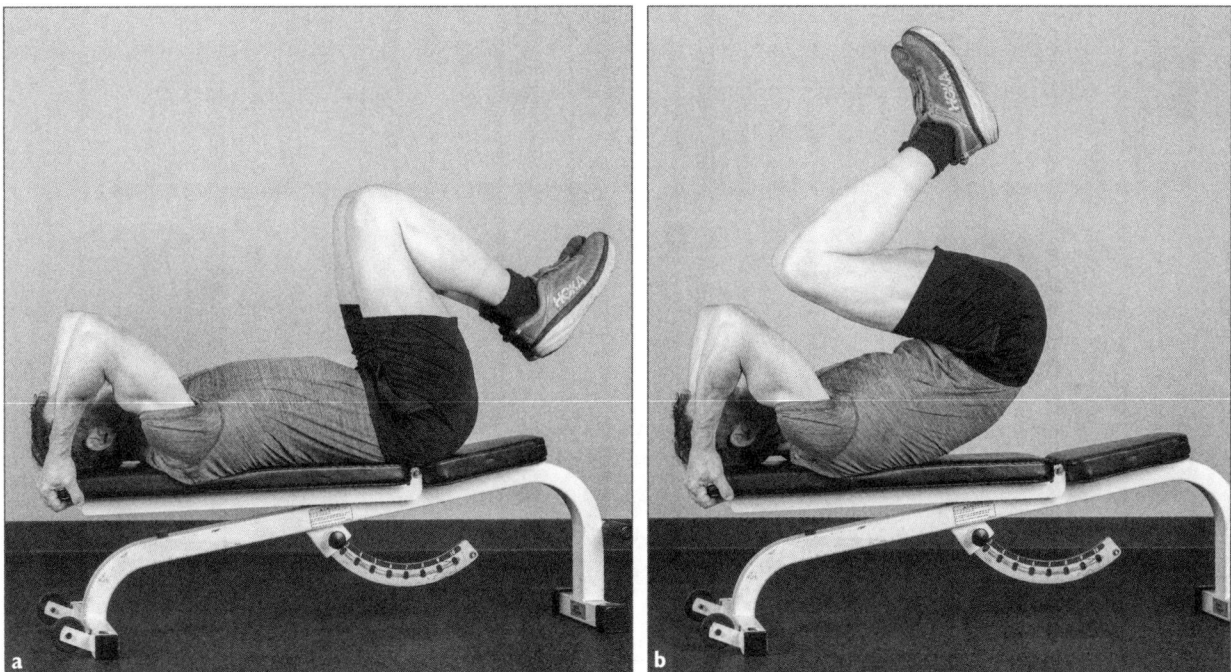

CHAD'S TAKE

Although there really aren't upper and lower abs, you will likely feel these in the lower abdominal area because you are pulling the pelvis up rather than curling the chest down. I prefer the bench because you can hold on tightly with your hands and provide a good anchor point. However, some might prefer to do this lying on an exercise mat or the floor. In that case, simply keep your arms down at your side for stability and use the same technique as the bench version.

Hanging Ab Raise

This is one of the toughest exercises I teach clients, and it's one of the toughest to do correctly. You'll need hanging abdominal slings to do these. Older gyms may have a hanging ab bench instead of slings. While I prefer slings, the bench or even hanging from a pull-up bar by your hands can work if your grip is strong enough.

The hip flexors are actually the muscles lifting the legs. The core muscles are bracing very hard to stabilize the pelvis in order to give the hip flexors a proper anchor with which to pull the legs up. Strong hip flexors are just as important as strong abs. If you want to go up a tall step or get into a high vehicle, you'll want strong hip flexors. However, if your abs are weak, you may not be able to stabilize the pelvis properly, and the hip flexors may "tug" on your lower back, causing pain. So only do the hanging ab raise if you already have strong abs.

INSTRUCTION

- Hang from a pull-up bar with an overhand grip, or use abdominal slings or a stand designed for hanging ab raises (figure *a*).
- Engage the core muscles and lift the knees of bent legs toward the chest (figure *b*).
- Lower the knees back down and repeat for 10 to 15 reps.

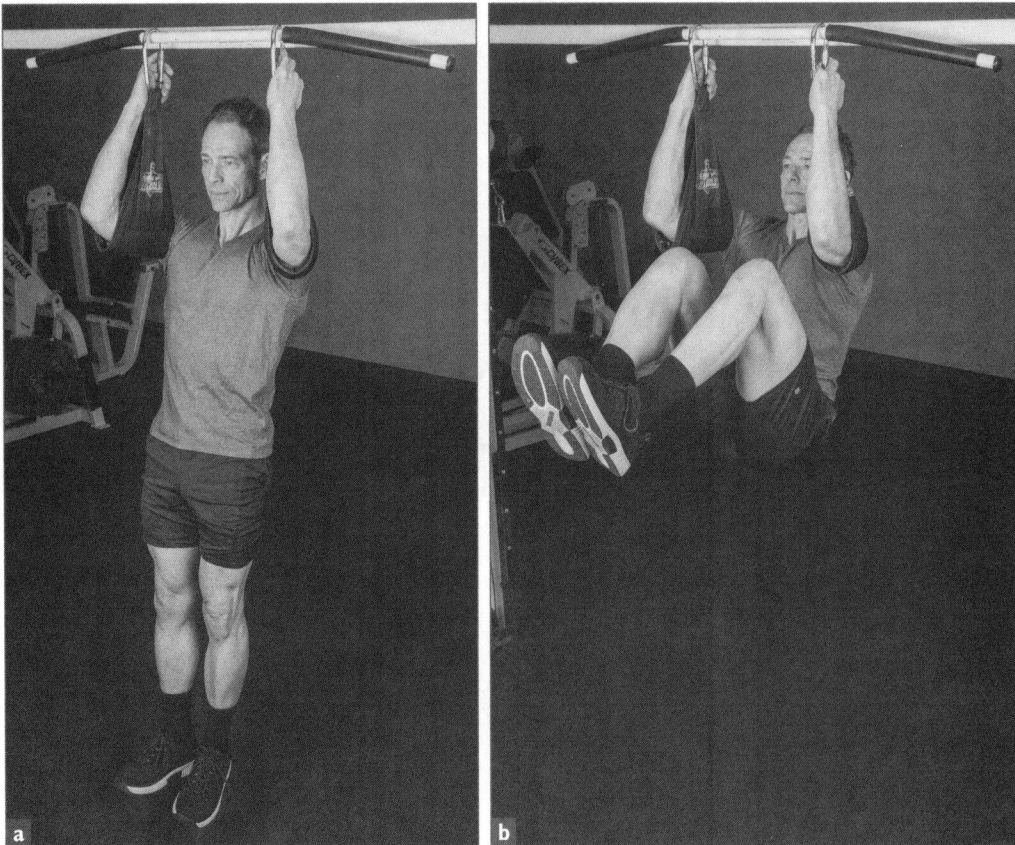

CHAD'S TAKE

The hanging ab raise is tough, and it's easy to butcher the form. Think of bracing the core and controlling the movement to prevent swinging on the way down. Eventually you'll also be able to bring the knees above parallel to the floor and even tilt the pelvis up as with the reverse crunch, but this is *very* advanced and should be performed only once you've established the requisite strength.

CHAPTER 9

Lower Body

From Tom Selleck's short shorts on *Magnum P.I.*, to Catherine Bach's "Daisy Dukes" on *The Dukes of Hazzard*, to every swimwear-clad cast member of *Baywatch*, Gen Xers have always appreciated a nice set of legs!

But strong legs aren't just for filling out Daisy Dukes, they help keep you alive and kicking! Similar to grip strength, leg strength is positively correlated with longevity. One study found that men and women whose thigh strength fell just one notch below average were 50–65 percent more likely to die during the 5-year follow up, even after the scientists accounted for differences in age, body fat, health problems, and activity level (Newman et al. 2006). They also found that muscle size didn't matter. So you don't have to have huge thighs, but they do need to be strong! Even younger generations should take heed to get strong. A study of more than one million Swedish teen conscripts found that the weakest 10 percent for leg strength faced a 32 percent higher risk of dying before age 55 and had nearly double the risk of a fatal heart event than their stronger peers (Ortega et al. 2012). Bottom line: skipping leg training is like expecting Magnum to chase crooks across Oahu with his red Ferrari up on blocks…you're not going to get very far.

Unfortunately, training legs is hard…you either love it or you hate it. In my experience, many women love it a bit too much and tend to overdo lower-body exercises, whilst many men hate it so badly they neglect to work their legs at all! And many active non-gymgoers assume their legs get enough work from walking, playing golf or tennis, yoga, and so on. Unfortunately, this isn't the case. Yes, those activities are great to do, but even professional runners know you still need dedicated strength training to achieve the best results.

Leg exercises do tend to be harder than upper-body work. They involve the largest muscles of the body and thus use heavier weights. Plus, these big muscles require a lot of oxygen when you're working them, so you'll typically get more out of breath than during upper-body exercises. And, yes, certain lower-body exercises such as leg extensions and calf raises have their own special burn you must experience to appreciate.

But the good news is that most trainees don't need a dedicated leg day. Instead, they should incorporate different leg exercises into their two or three days a week of full-body training. However, those with competitive aspirations (bodybuilding or powerlifting) may find dedicated leg days useful.

It can be difficult to know just what to do, though. There is a big range between "my legs get enough work being on my feet all day" and "I couldn't walk right for three days after my killer leg day." We have lots of leg muscles and thus lots of lower-body exercises to choose from, so it can feel overwhelming. But those exercises can be categorized a number of ways:

- Location: thighs, calves, hips, glutes
- Function: extension or flexion
- Muscle: quadriceps, hamstrings, gastrocnemius, soleus, gluteus maximus, gluteus medius
- Dominance of muscle group: hip dominant versus quad dominant
- Number of legs working: unilateral (one) versus bilateral (two)
- Number of muscles/joints involved: compound versus isolation
- Plane of motion: sagittal, frontal, transverse

Overwhelming indeed!

The programs I use with clients and share in this book incorporate all these ideas to a degree, but I try to simplify how to go about grouping and selecting exercises to use and how often to do them. The truth is there is no must-do exercise. For instance, as great an exercise as the barbell squat is, I no longer do it—at age 56, with osteoarthritis in both knees and a history of Baker's cysts, my knees just don't do well after squatting. Plus, I don't want to hasten the need for knee replacement surgery, something many 50-somethings have already dealt with or are well on their way toward.

So if an exercise causes you undue pain, or it just doesn't feel right, a suitable work-around exists. Take your time and experiment with different exercises and find out what works for you. We are playing the long game after 50, and no single exercise or workout is going to make us, but it could break us. As the Grail Knight said in *Indiana Jones and the Last Crusade*, "You must choose, but choose wisely."

Calves are one area where I give the client some leeway. Some people genetically have huge calves and already have a hard time buying boots or trouble wearing jeans and simply don't want to make their calves bigger. I completely understand, and it's not a hill I'm willing to die on.

This doesn't mean there wouldn't be other benefits (strength, injury prevention) if they did work their calves, but it's their choice. So, if this is you, you have my permission to skip calf training. But most of you should at least do some standing calf raises and probably anterior tibialis work, too. No matter how large your calves are naturally, it's a good idea to take them through their full range of motion regularly to stay flexible and supple.

The exercises in this chapter are not an encyclopedia of every leg exercise; they are the exercises I use most often in my own workouts and especially with older trainees. I find them easiest to learn and execute but varied enough to work all the muscles of the lower body.

The following categories make sense for how I see leg exercises. Some might say that a certain exercise belongs in a different category, but all of them are worth experimenting with regardless of name or category—like my client who calls Swiss ball leg curls "crampy crampersons." So play around with these, and rename them if you like, but as Nike inspired us years ago, *just do it*.

QUAD-DOMINANT EXERCISES

When working the muscles of the upper thigh, an easy way to categorize exercises is by the muscle group being focused on. *Quad-dominant* simply means that the exercise tends to work the quadriceps muscles on the front of the thigh more than the glutes and hamstrings on the back of the thigh.

This could mean a quad isolation like machine leg extensions, but it more often refers to multi-joint exercises that work muscles other than the quads, but the quad is still the dominant muscle being worked. In this chapter I've grouped the "larger" multi-joint quad-dominant exercises, multi-joint hip-dominant exercises, combination quad-hip exercises, and quad and hamstring isolation exercises.

Goblet Squat

The goblet squat is the first squat I teach new clients. If someone has never squatted before, it's far easier to learn the proper form using a goblet squat than a barbell back squat. Its name comes from the shape the arms and dumbbell make when holding one end of the dumbbell with two hands at chest level.

INSTRUCTION

- Stand with your feet shoulder-width apart, toes slightly turned out.
- Grab a dumbbell from one end with a hand on each side so the weight is resting on your palms (figure a), basically forming the shape of a goblet with your arms and hands.
- Lower your body, keeping your back straight and your chest up.
- Squat down as far as is comfortable or until your thighs are parallel to the ground (figure b).
- Drive evenly through the balls of the feet and heels back up to the starting position.

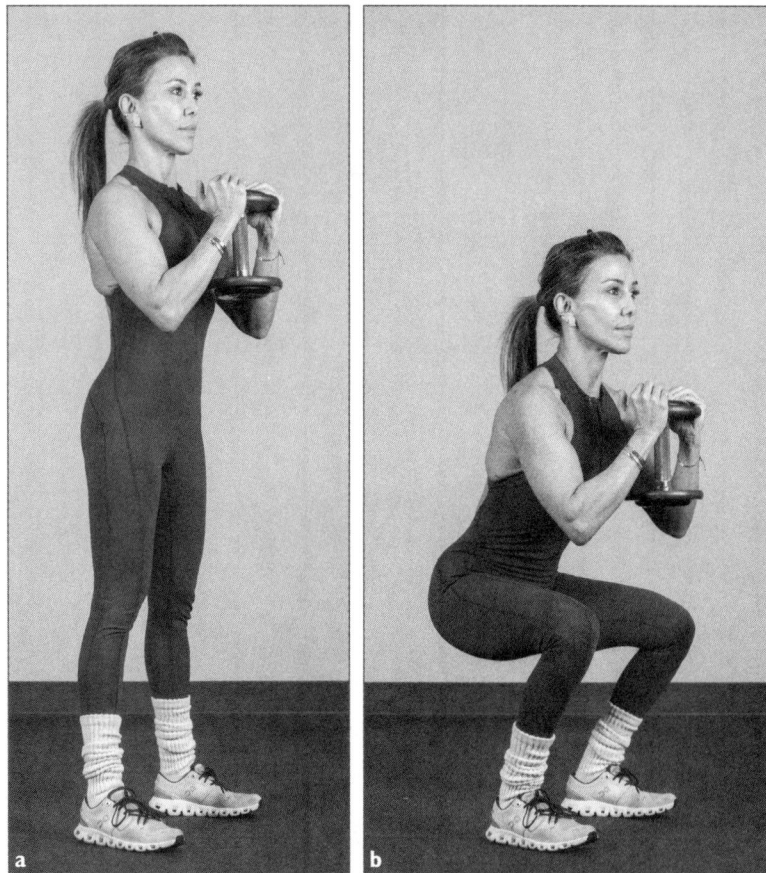

CHAD'S TAKE

As I said earlier, the goblet squat is much easier to learn than the traditional barbell back squat and barbell front squat. And for the over-50 crowd with shoulder or lower back issues, goblet squats tend to be much more comfortable than holding a barbell on the shoulders. Even with very strong clients, I'll often use the combo of a dumbbell and weighted vest rather than use barbell variations.

Bulgarian Split Squat

Why Bulgaria gets the credit for this exercise is beyond me, but you may have also heard it called a rear-foot elevated split squat, which is quite a mouthful. You can think of this as a one-legged squat even though the position more closely resembles a lunge.

INSTRUCTION

- Stand with your back to a bench or low platform or box.
- Place one foot on the bench behind you. The knee of the rear leg should be slightly behind the hip (figure a).
- Lower your body until your front thigh is parallel to the ground (figure b). You should feel a bit of a stretch in the hip flexors of the rear leg when going down during the exercise.
- Drive evenly through the balls of the feet and heels back up to the starting position. Start with your weaker side, then repeat on the stronger side for the same number of reps.

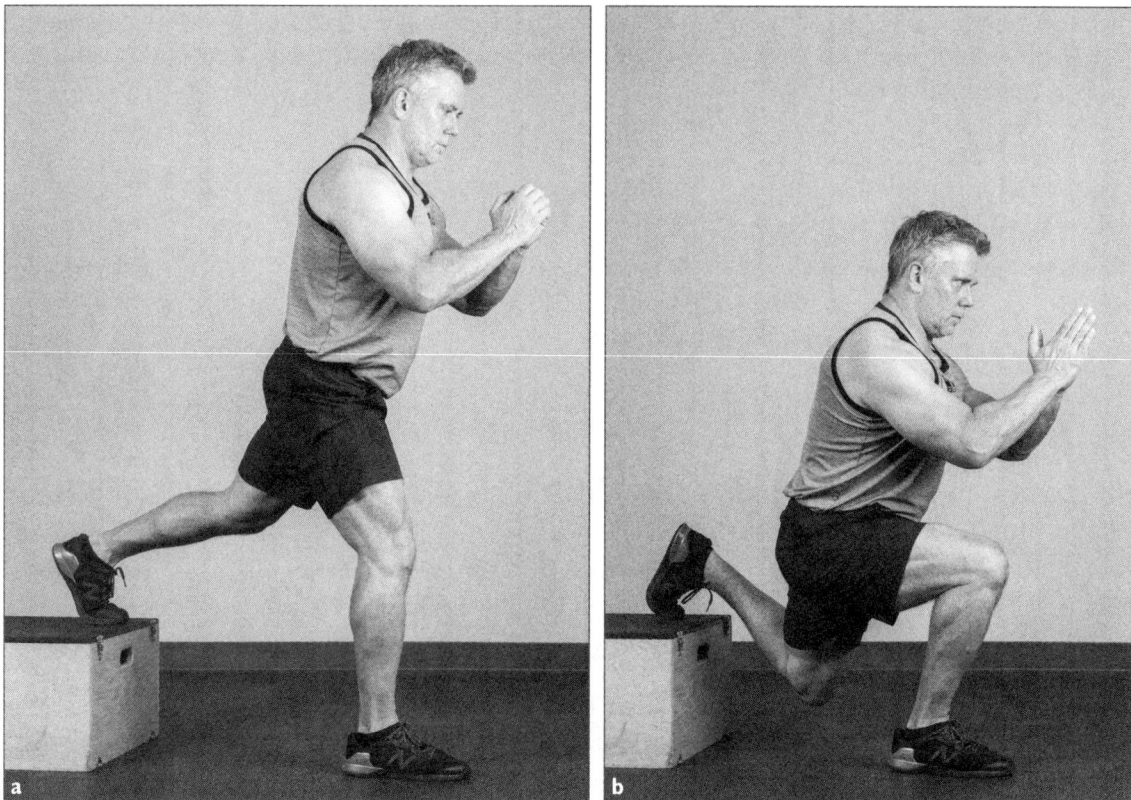

CHAD'S TAKE

The Bulgarian split squat is a great, albeit challenging, unilateral quad exercise. Newer trainees may prefer to start with the rear foot on the floor (split squat), rather than elevated. This version will likely feel easier to balance and control than the Bulgarian version. However, if you like the exercise, you'll probably want to add an external load by wearing a weighted vest or by holding dumbbells at your sides. I'm not a huge fan of using a barbell on your back with this because if you lose your balance, the damage to you (and the gym) will likely be greater.

Leg Press

The leg press might be the most ubiquitous machine in commercial gyms. Various types exist, from plate-loaded to selectorized weight stacks, some machines lying flat, others at a 45-degree angle, some with a moving foot plate, and others where the feet are fixed and the upper body moves the machine kind of like a lying squat.

Although I prefer to do mostly squats, deadlifts, and lunges with clients, the leg press is a great option. First, you can get very strong without having to put a big load on your spine. Second, the technique is straightforward and easier to master than the free-weight or body-weight movements.

INSTRUCTION

- Sit in the leg press machine with your back against the pad and your feet on the foot plate about shoulder-width apart with toes angled out slightly, similar to your squat stance.
- Push up on the foot plate and remove the safety supports (figure *a*).
- Lower the weight as far as comfortable or until your knees are at a 90-degree angle (figure *b*). Be careful not to bring the lower back and hips off the back pad by trying to stretch too far at the bottom.
- Drive evenly through the balls of the feet and heels back up to the starting position.

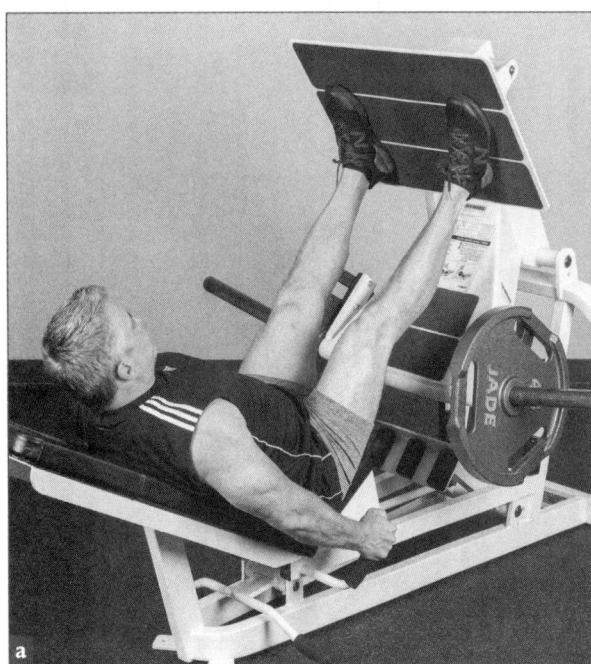

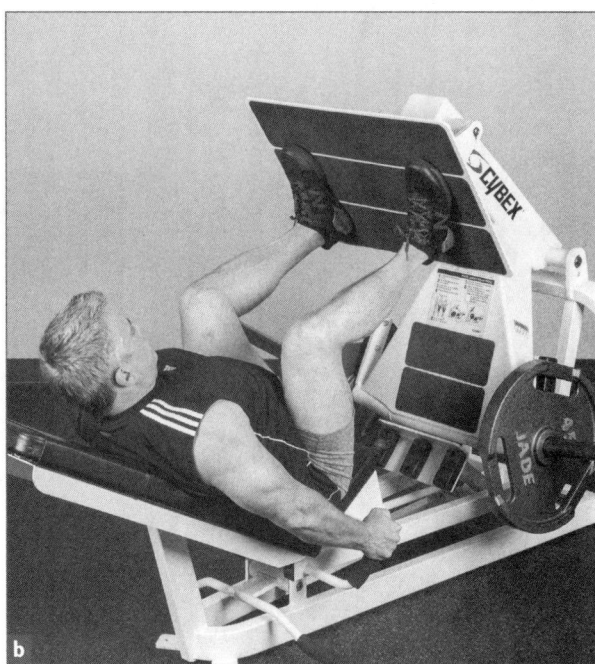

CHAD'S TAKE

I tend to start clients with multiplanar bodyweight exercises such as step-ups, bodyweight squats, bridges, and side shuffles before using the leg press. It's too easy to lift too heavy too soon without first strengthening all the muscles that move, stabilize, and assist motion in all planes. It's a great exercise and a fine choice in rotation with the exercises I mentioned, just don't make it your only leg exercise.

HIP-DOMINANT EXERCISES

As you may have guessed, hip-dominant exercises focus more on the glutes and hamstrings than the quads. A common descriptor of many of these exercises is a *hip hinge*. We are focused more on the actions of the glutes (and to a lesser degree the hamstrings) on the hip than we are about the quads extending the knees. Exercises where the knees stay in a fairly fixed position and the hips are flexing and extending will isolate the glutes and hamstrings. A good visual I like to use for the hip hinge harkens back to the '70s and '80s. How many of you had a great aunt or granny who had one of those weird glass "drinking birds" with the top hat in their tchotchke collection? If you remember, the head would go down and the butt would come up and back in unison, while the back and legs were eternally straight. That's basically your hip hinge.

Hex-Bar Deadlift

First, a note on deadlifts and breathing: As a powerlifter, I prefer to hold my breath from the moment right before I lift the bar off the ground until it is back down on the ground. This maintains a great deal of intra-abdominal pressure while under such a heavy load. However, most recreational lifters find this difficult and can even get lightheaded or pass out. You can maintain a similar pressure by doing *pursed lips breathing*, where you exhale slowly under pressure through pursed lips as you lift the weight. Then either rebrace and set the weight down or inhale again at the top of the movement and rebrace before setting it down. Find the method that works best for you to maintain core bracing and not get lightheaded.

INSTRUCTION

- Stand with feet hip-width apart and toes slightly turned out.
- Place the loaded hex bar on the ground in front of you.
- Keeping the chest up, push the hips back, bend down, and grip the bar using a neutral grip standard to the hex bar (figure *a*).
- Inhale and brace your core. While holding your breath, drive through your heels, push your hips forward, and stand up straight (figure *b*).
- Lower the hex bar back down to the ground under control.

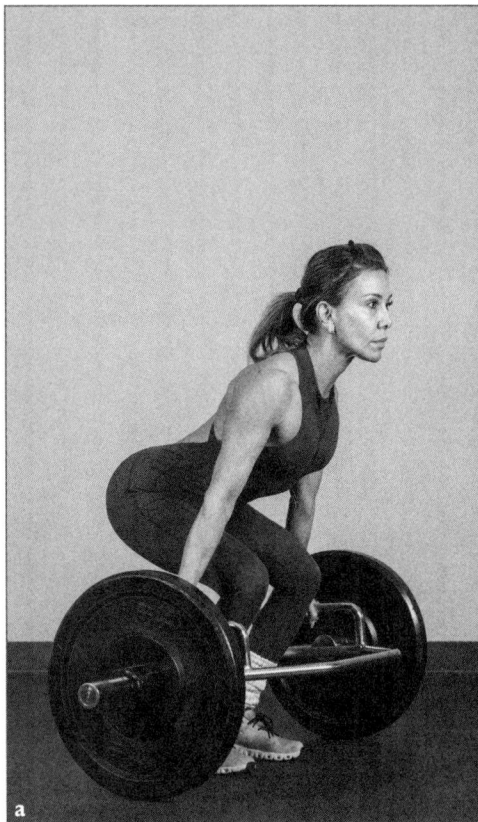

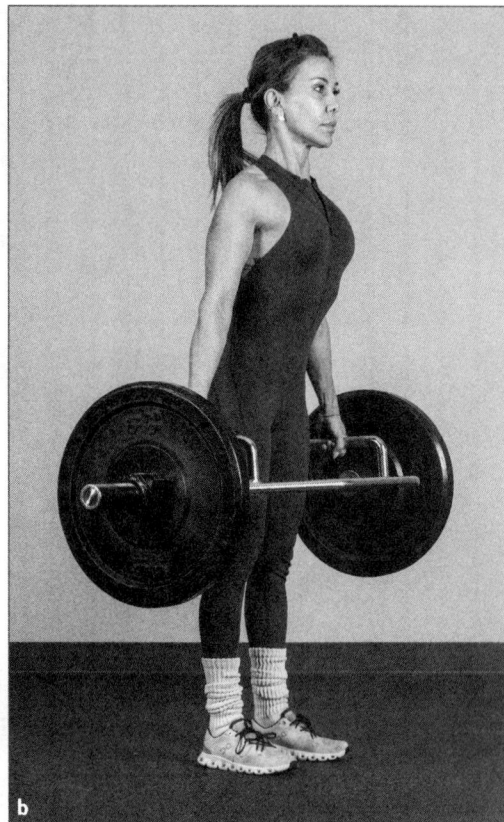

CHAD'S TAKE

I much prefer that everyone use the hex bar instead of a traditional barbell deadlift unless they are a competitive powerlifter or have no hex bar available. The position of the body within the center of the weights with a hex bar is much safer than having the weights in front of the body's center of gravity as with a straight barbell.

Kettlebell Swing

The kettlebell swing is a great exercise to develop power (think strength plus speed), which diminishes as we age. Done properly, it is a textbook example of a hip hinge. But beware—the dynamic stretch you get in the glutes and hamstrings can make you pretty sore if you haven't been doing these.

INSTRUCTION

- Stand with feet shoulder-width apart, toes slightly turned out. Place a kettlebell between your feet and slightly in front of your body.
- Grab the handle of the kettlebell with both hands, palms facing down.
- Hinge at the hips and swing the kettlebell back between your legs (figure *a*).
- Drive through your hips, pushing them forward and swinging the kettlebell up between about hip and chest level; do not lift with the arms, allow hip drive only to dictate the height of the swing (figure *b*).

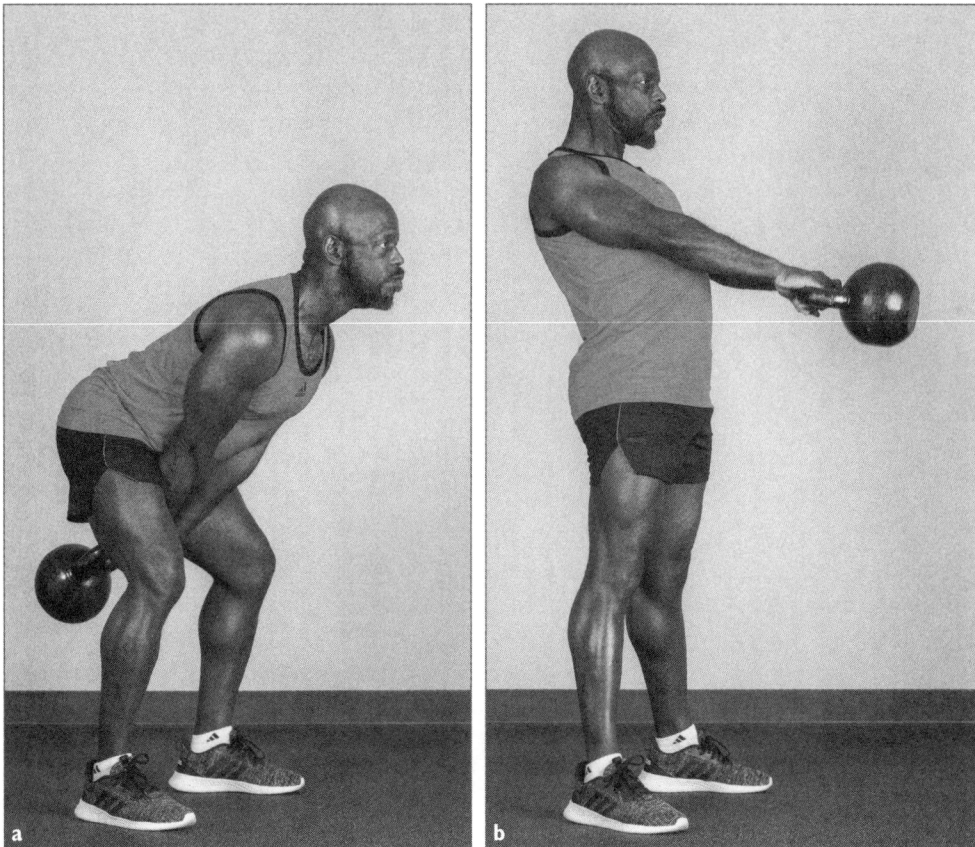

CHAD'S TAKE

The are a few alternatives to the traditional kettlebell swing. Some people like to use a kettlebell in each hand, but I find the extrawide stance required to be quite uncomfortable. Others like to hold onto the kettlebell with one hand; this can be OK if you only have light kettlebells and don't need two hands to control the bell, but you'll want to do the same number of reps on each side. There is also the American kettlebell swing, but I don't like this one because it has you swing the bell all the way overhead, which is unnecessary to work the hip hinge and is potentially dangerous.

COMBINATION QUAD AND HIP EXERCISES

I call these combo exercises because they aren't purely quad dominant, like squats, or hip dominant, like deadlifts. These exercises work a little bit of everything and also happen to be unilateral exercises, which benefits balanced development.

I consider these "big" exercises like squats and deadlifts, and they are staples of all my programs. As such, I use them in place of those exercises, not in addition to them. If I desire added leg work beyond a quad, hip, or combo exercise, I'll choose one of the specific exercises later in this chapter rather than multiple big leg exercises in one workout.

Reverse Lunge

The reverse lunge is my favorite unilateral leg exercise and the first one I teach after the step-up. The balance and coordination needed are a bit less with this lunge than with a regular lunge and the step-up, so it is easier to learn and easier to start adding external loads with a weighted vest or dumbbells. As with all unilateral exercises, start with the weaker side first and match those reps on the stronger side.

INSTRUCTION

- Stand straight with your feet hip-width apart and your hands in front of you (figure *a*).
- Take a step back with your left foot and lower your body until your right knee is bent (aim for 90 degrees) and your left knee hovers just above the floor (figure *b*). Your back should be straight but with a slight forward lean over the front foot. It is OK if your right knee goes beyond your right toes, but it shouldn't be painful.
- Push back up to the starting position by driving your front foot into the floor.
- Complete all repetitions on one leg, then switch sides and repeat for the same number of reps.

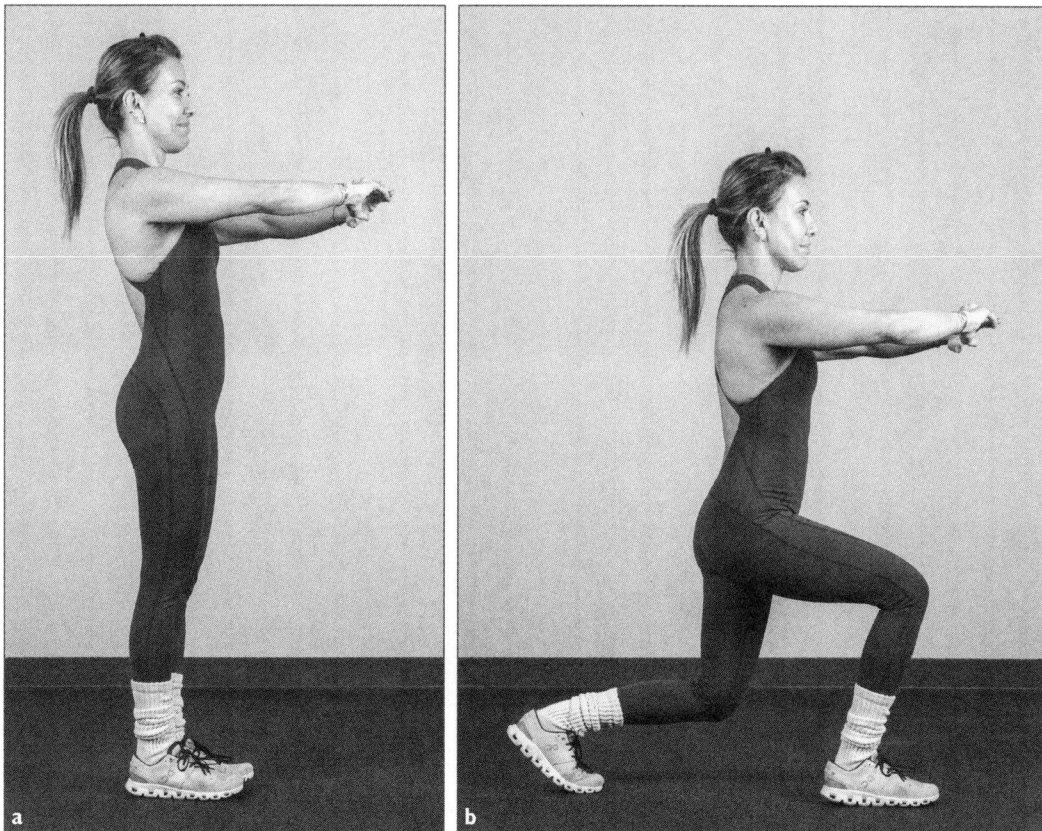

CHAD'S TAKE

If you need to make the exercise a bit easier, you can alternate sides rather than doing one side at a time. Alternating sides allows each leg to briefly rest while the other side works. It's not a huge difference but is a great option if necessary. I also like to do this lunge with the rear foot on a furniture slider (or exercise slider) as it cues you to keep the weight forward on the front foot. Also, I prefer to bring the arm opposite the front leg forward and vice versa, like a running motion.

Lunge

Another great unilateral combination leg exercise, the lunge not only works all the muscles of the legs, but promotes balance, coordination, and flexibility, something all older trainees should aim for.

INSTRUCTION

- Stand straight with your feet hip-width apart and your hands in front of you (figure a).
- Step forward with your right foot and lower your body until your right knee is bent (aim for 90 degrees) and your left knee hovers just above the floor (figure b). Keep your back straight but with a forward lean over the front (right) foot.
- Drive back up to the starting position through the ball of your right foot.
- Repeat for desired reps on one side, then repeat on the other.

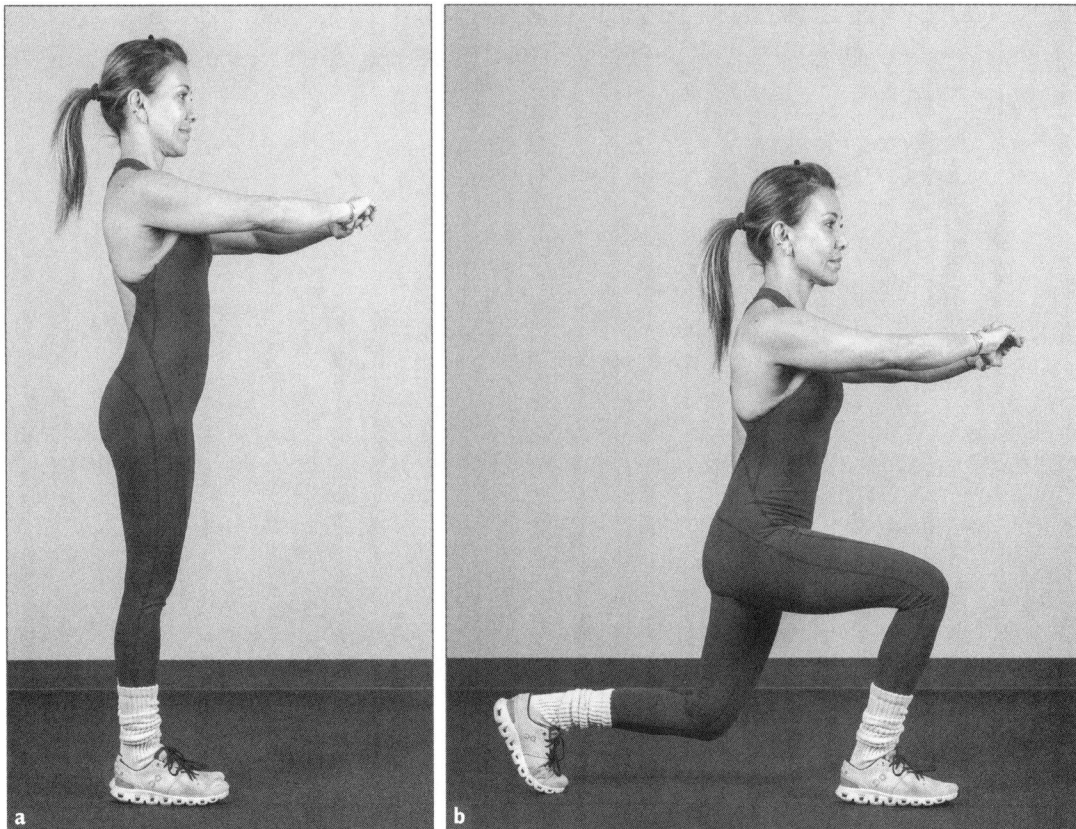

CHAD'S TAKE

I like the lunge to be more powerful and explosive than the reverse lunge. Think of pushing the ground away from you to power up to the start position. I don't do the running motion with my arms like I use on the reverse lunge—I find it beneficial to keep my arms down and use them for balance as needed. The walking lunge is another great variation if your gym has the open space. Instead of driving back as on a regular lunge, you'll continue to drive forward, alternating legs for the desired number of repetitions.

Step-Up

The step-up is the first exercise I show every new client. It gives me a picture of strength, balance, coordination, and athleticism in one quick bite. Most clients start with a 12-inch box, but some may need to start with a 6-inch or even a 3-inch box. Also, if possible, I progress to (or even start with) a slightly more advanced version where I start with the hand opposite the foot on the box in the air. As you step up, the arms switch position and the knee of the leg not on the box gets lifted until the thigh is roughly parallel to the ground. This takes more balance and coordination than the basic version.

INSTRUCTION

- Stand upright facing an exercise box or similar sturdy surface. Place the foot of the nondominant side on the box. Keep the arms in front of you (figure *a*).
- Press the foot on the box down into the box as you straighten that leg (figure *b*). You may place the opposite foot on the box for balance.
- Slowly lower and return to the start position. Repeat all repetitions on one leg, then switch legs and repeat for the same number of reps.

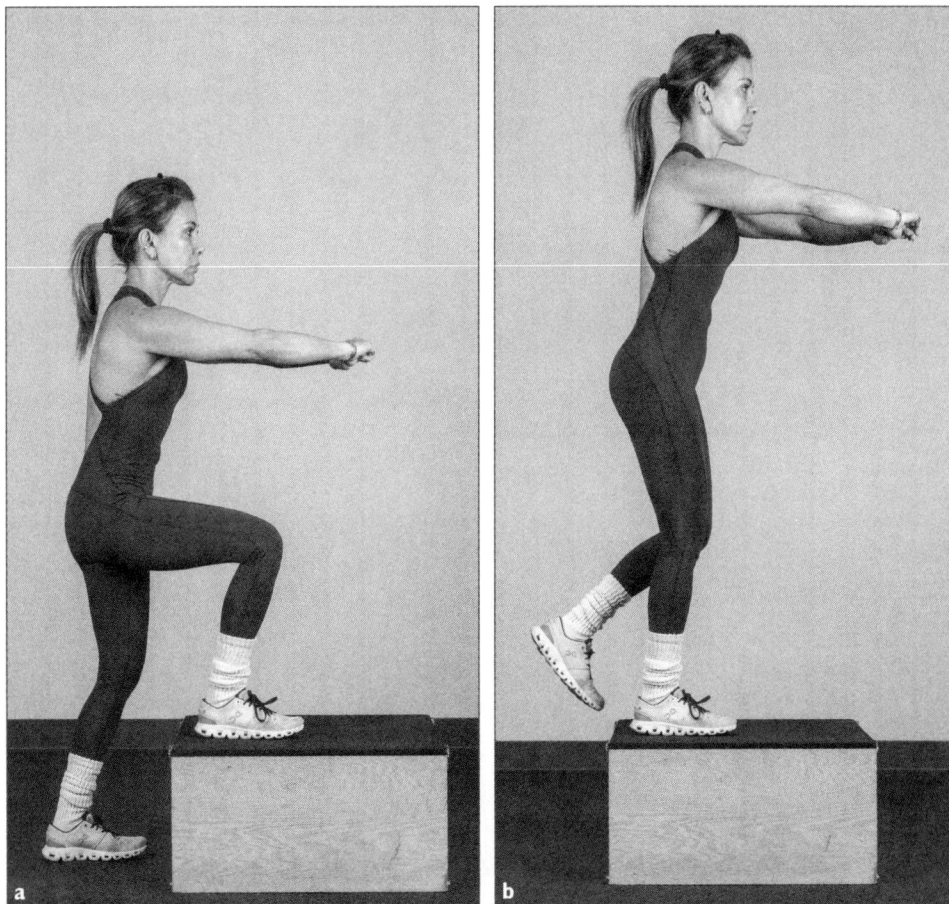

CHAD'S TAKE

This is another exercise I especially love for mature trainees because it requires strength, balance, and coordination. Clients who get proficient at these are "ready for Machu Picchu," as I tell them, because they won't be limited in their travels by lack of strength and athleticism.

GLUTE-SPECIFIC EXERCISES

Glute-specific is a bit of a misnomer because there are about 17 muscles of the gluteal and hip region, and you will never completely isolate the glute muscles. However, the term is an easy way to differentiate the "smaller" exercises of this region.

Hip Thrust or Glute Bridge

You've likely come across this exercise through one of its common names. The hip thrust has gained a huge following, primarily thanks to the work of Bret Contreras, aka the Glute Guy. It's become so popular, in fact, that multiple gym-equipment manufacturers have come up with machine versions of this exercise. If your gym has one, use it. Otherwise, if you need to add external load to your hip thrusts, you'll need to use a padded barbell on your hip bones.

INSTRUCTION

- Lie on an exercise mat with knees bent and arms down at the sides.
- Plant your feet on the ground, hip-width apart (figure a).
- Drive through your heels, lifting your hips up toward the ceiling (figure b).
- Lower your hips to the starting position.

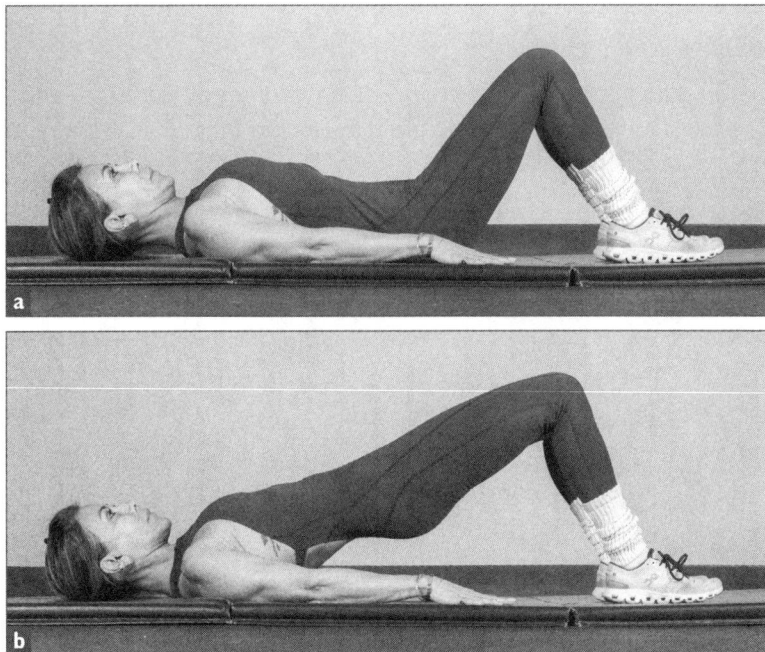

CHAD'S TAKE

This is great for the glutes, and there are several variations I employ. I like to add an exercise band around the knees to get a little more outer hip work without external load. You can also try it elevated with your back on a bench. I prefer the back-on-bench version when adding external load because it's easier to balance at the top of the movement. I leave the exercise band out when adding external load because it gets a bit cumbersome to deal with while also controlling a barbell on your hips.

Banded Side Shuffle

There are so few exercises that work the hips in the frontal plane that the banded side shuffle is a staple of my programs. It is far more comfortable and effective using modern wide fabric elastic bands compared with latex rubber band options. Thinner rubber bands probably won't provide enough resistance and could even break, while even thicker bands tend to pinch the skin and/or pull leg hair if wearing shorts. I personally do not use rubber bands for this exercise, but if it's all you have available, you can try using them knowing the caveats I mentioned above.

INSTRUCTION

- Stand upright with your knees flexed and your feet shoulder-width apart. Place a rubber or fabric exercise band above the knees (figure a).
- Step sideways to stretch the band out fully (figure b).
- Lift the foot of the trailing leg and resist the pull of the band, allowing the feet to return to the shoulder-width starting position.
- Do the desired number of steps then repeat in the other direction to return to where you started. You can also do these in place by alternating sides back and forth rather than shuffling across the gym.

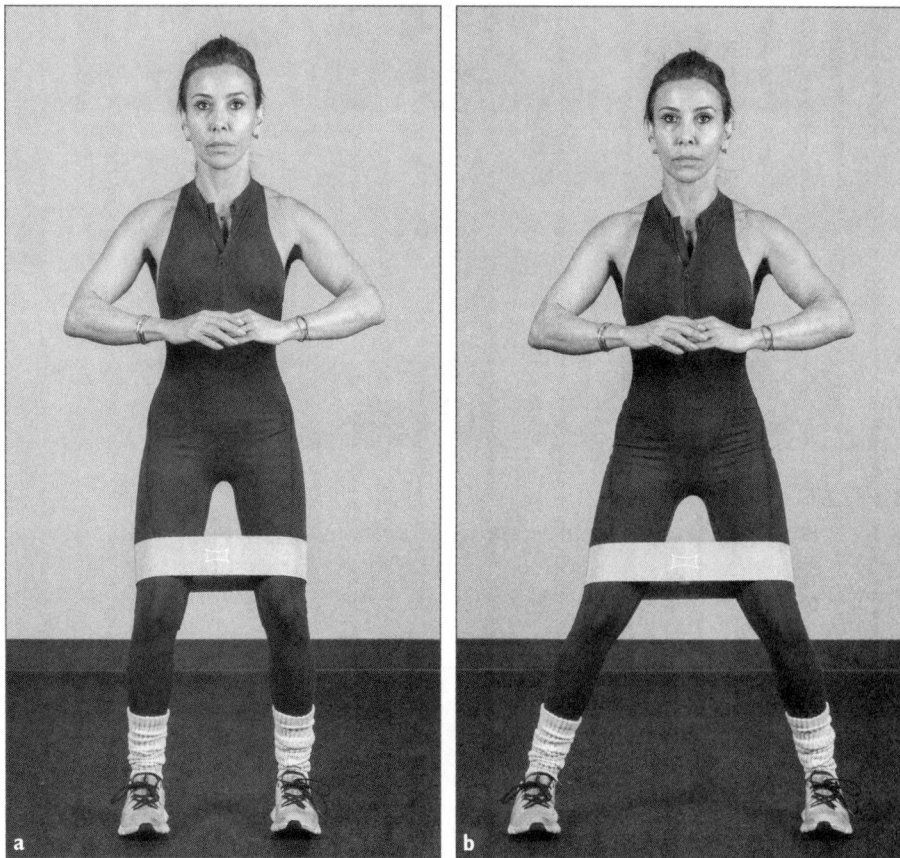

CHAD'S TAKE

I find this exercise especially helpful to avoid the "old man butt" that many older trainees are stricken with. Get ready to feel the burn!

HAMSTRING-SPECIFIC EXERCISES

I find that clients have a better time connecting to their hamstrings using hamstring-specific exercises, so I include them liberally in my programs.

Lying Leg Curl

The lying leg curl has been around in some form for decades. Most newer machines have an angled bench that allows you to bend at the hips while lying face down, which is far more comfortable (and likely safer on the lower back) than the old-school version with a completely flat pad to lie on. If your gym has one of these old machines, do a different hamstring exercise.

INSTRUCTION

- Lie prone (face down) on the leg curl machine and adjust the machine lever to fit your height. The pad of the leg lever should be on the back of your legs, above the heel but under the calves.
- Keeping your torso flat on the bench, ensure that your legs are fully stretched and grab the side handles of the machine (figure *a*).
- Curl your legs up as far as possible, aiming to touch the pad to the back of the thighs (figure *b*).
- Slowly lower the legs back to the initial position.

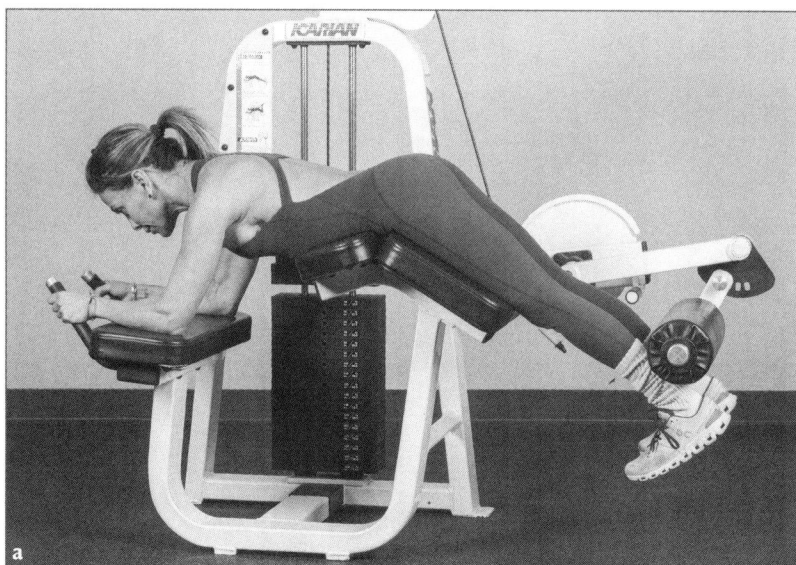

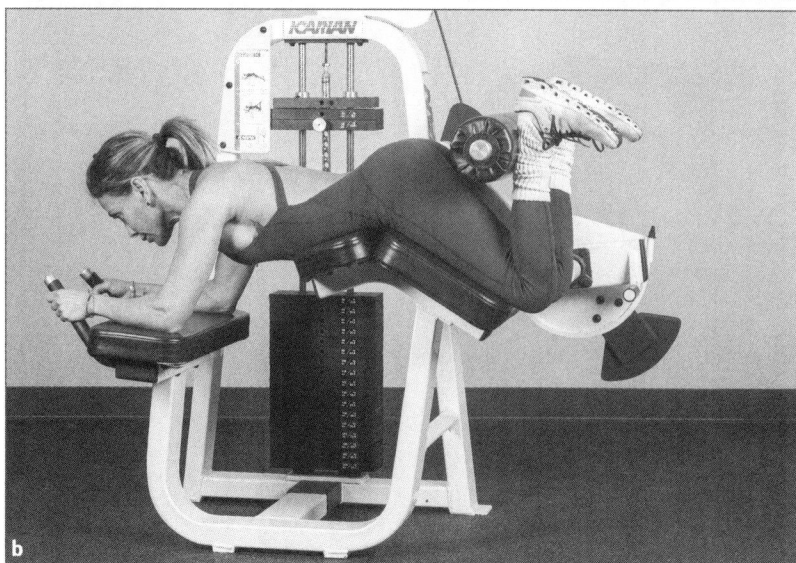

CHAD'S TAKE

Although seated leg curls have become more popular than the lying version in recent years, not all gyms have the seated version. The lying leg curl is a fine substitute, as long as it has an angled pad to lie on. I like to lift my thighs off the pad at the top of the movement to create more hip extension and get a full contraction of the hamstrings. I dorsiflex the ankle on these, too.

Seated Leg Curl

The seated leg curl is a staple in most of my programs. It's a great hamstring-specific exercise and a good choice for those who aren't able to do exercises like the Swiss ball leg curl because of hamstring weakness.

INSTRUCTION

- Adjust the machine lever to fit your height and sit on the machine with your back against the back pad.
- Position the lower leg pad so it's resting just above your heels, and adjust the thigh pad so it's snug against your thighs. Grasp the side handles on the machine (figure *a*).
- Pull the leg lever as far as possible to the back of your thighs by flexing at the knees, while keeping your torso stationary and your back against the back pad (figure *b*).
- Slowly return the lever to the initial position, taking care not to touch the weight stack between repetitions.

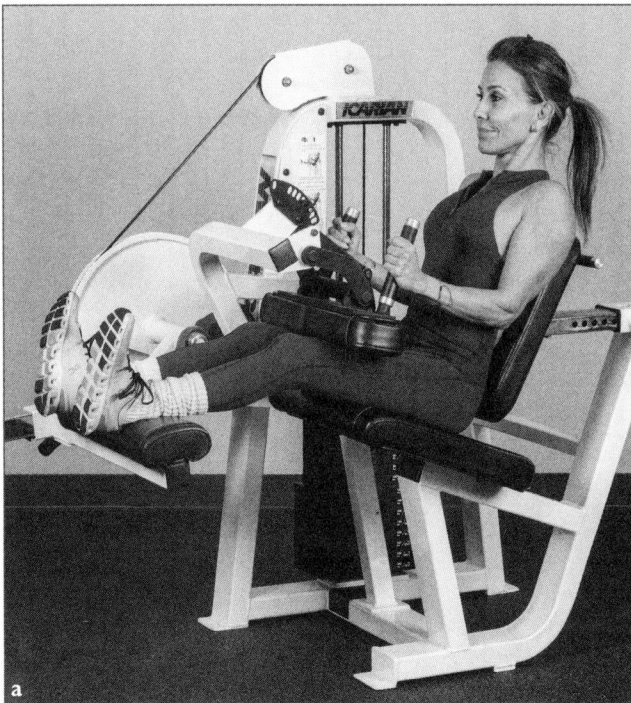

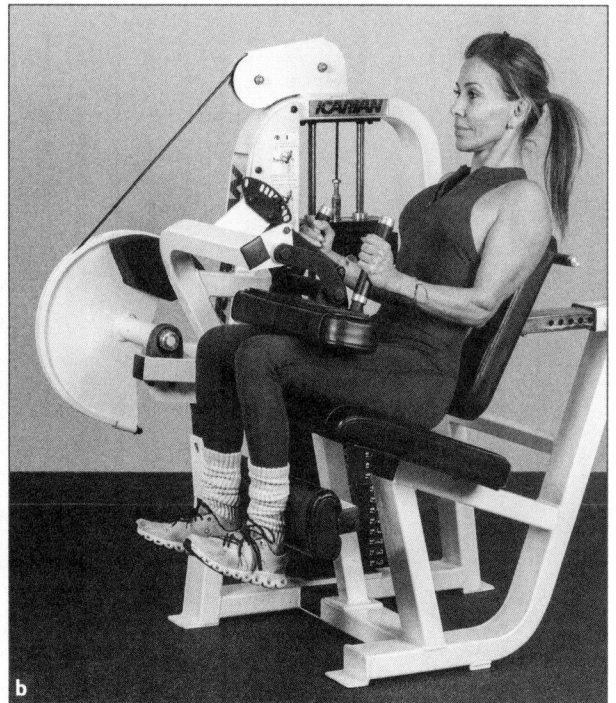

CHAD'S TAKE

I love the seated leg curl. It tends to be more comfortable for more clients than the lying leg curl, and it provides a great training stimulus for the hamstrings. I like to keep my ankle dorsiflexed (toe pulled toward shin) during the exercise to minimize the assistance of the gastrocnemius muscle of the calves by keeping it stretched during the movement.

Swiss Ball Leg Curl

The Swiss ball leg curl is perhaps my favorite hamstring exercise, especially for older trainees, because it allows for both knee flexion and hip extension for a full contraction of the hamstrings. It can create a massive contraction, and many a client has felt a hamstring cramp when first doing this exercise, so beware.

INSTRUCTION

- Lie flat on your back on an exercise mat. Keep your arms at your sides, palms flat against the floor for stability. (Do *not* use the arms to lift your body, however.)
- Place your heels just past the top of the Swiss ball so the Achilles tendon is on top of the ball, legs extended and feet together or slightly apart.
- Lift your hips off the ground by pressing down through your lower legs on the Swiss ball and engaging your glutes and hamstrings. Your body should form a straight line from your shoulders to your heels (figure *a*).
- From this position, bend your knees to roll the Swiss ball toward your body, keeping your hips elevated (figure *b*).
- Extend your knees to roll the ball back out to the starting position while maintaining the elevated hip position.

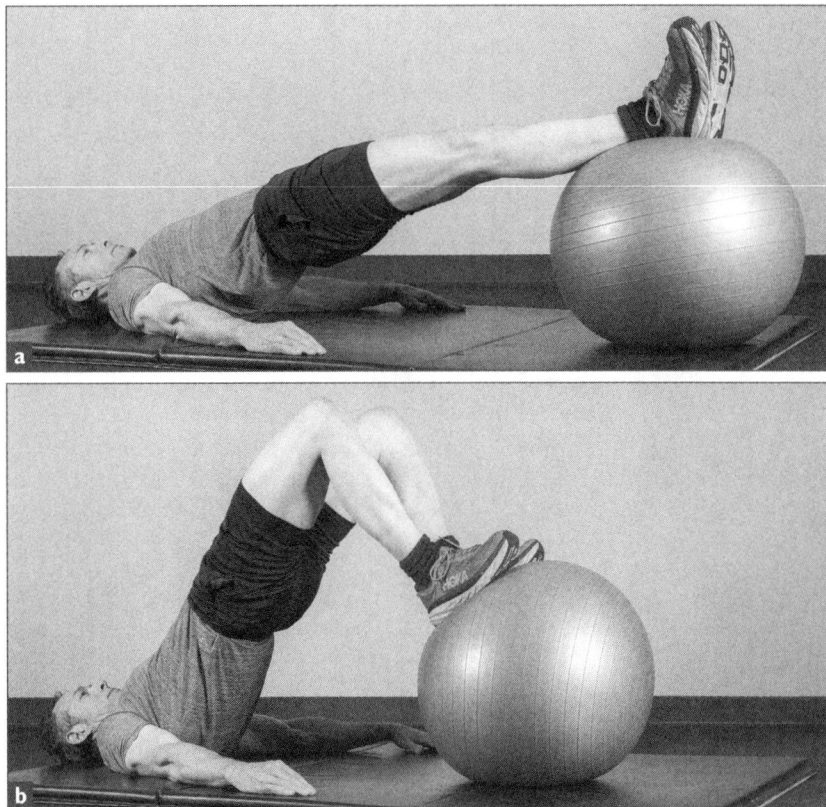

CHAD'S TAKE

Older trainees often complain that their hamstrings feel tight. The more likely reality is that the hamstrings are weak, and the nervous system is protecting them by not allowing too big a stretch. Nothing strengthens the hamstrings like exercises that do both knee flexion and hip extension. Another variation I like is with the feet on furniture sliders (or exercise sliders) rather than on a Swiss ball.

Romanian Deadlift

The Romanian deadlift is a great hamstring exercise but puts an extreme amount of tension on the hamstrings, so start with very light weight. Make sure to use a slow, controlled motion on the stretch and avoid "bouncing" out of the stretch position. This is also known as a stiff-legged deadlift. There is also a straight-leg deadlift, which uses a straight, locked knee rather than a straight, stiff but unlocked knee. This is mainly semantics, so do what feels best for you and your knees.

INSTRUCTION

- Stand with feet hip-width apart and toes slightly turned out with knees straight but not locked.
- Hold the barbell with an overhand grip, hands shoulder-width apart (figure *a*).
- Hinge at the hips and push the butt back while keeping your back straight and your chest up, lowering the barbell down the thighs and shins until you feel a stretch in your hamstrings (figure *b*).
- Drive back up to the starting position by contracting the glutes and hamstrings.

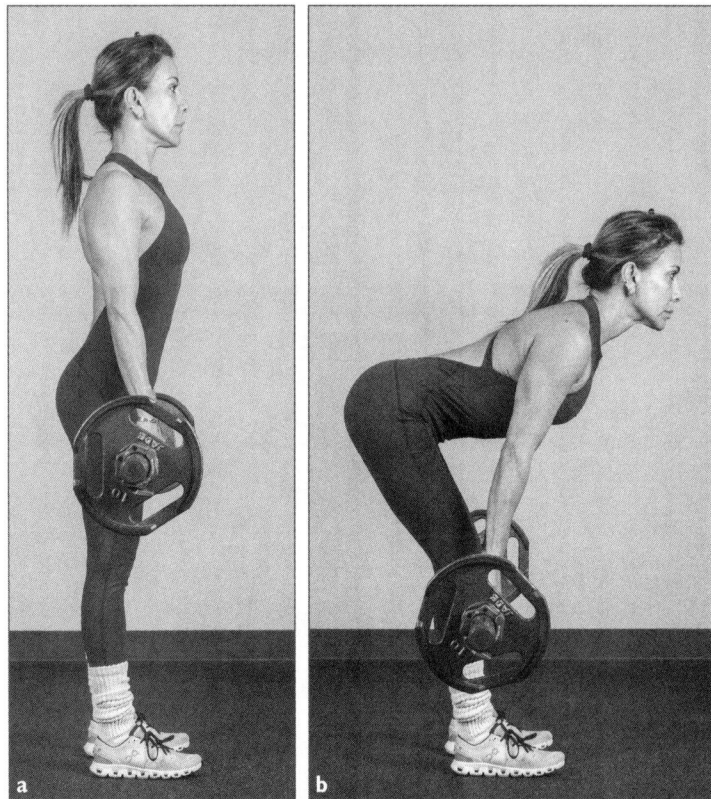

CHAD'S TAKE

This is another great exercise to keep older hamstrings strong and flexible. Feel free to use wrist straps to aid your grip if you get strong on these and need them. While I consider these a hamstring exercise, they really are hamstrings and glutes.

QUAD-SPECIFIC EXERCISES

There are a few quad-specific exercises out there, but I only include leg extensions regularly in my programs. I typically rely on multi-joint quad-dominant and combo exercises to work the quads. However, some trainees with arthritic knees may find they are able to do leg extensions when they can't do squats or other moves pain-free.

Leg Extension Machine

The leg extension machine is special. I still remember the first time I used one of the original Nautilus machines in high school in the early '80s. Holy crap, this exercise will make your quads burn like no other. It is one of the only exercises that isolates the quads well, if that's what you're looking for.

INSTRUCTION

- Adjust the seat back to fit your height and sit on the machine with your back against the back pad.
- Position the leg pad so it rests just above your foot against your lower leg but not too high up on the shin. Grasp the side handles on the machine (figure *a*).
- Extend the knees to raise the leg pad until your legs are straight with knees fully extended, keeping your torso stationary and your back against the back pad (figure *b*).
- Slowly return the pad to the initial position, taking care not to touch the weight stack between repetitions.

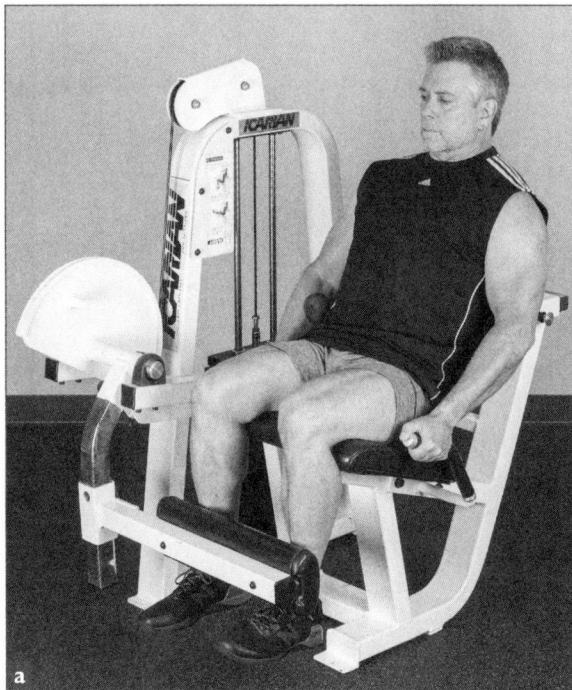

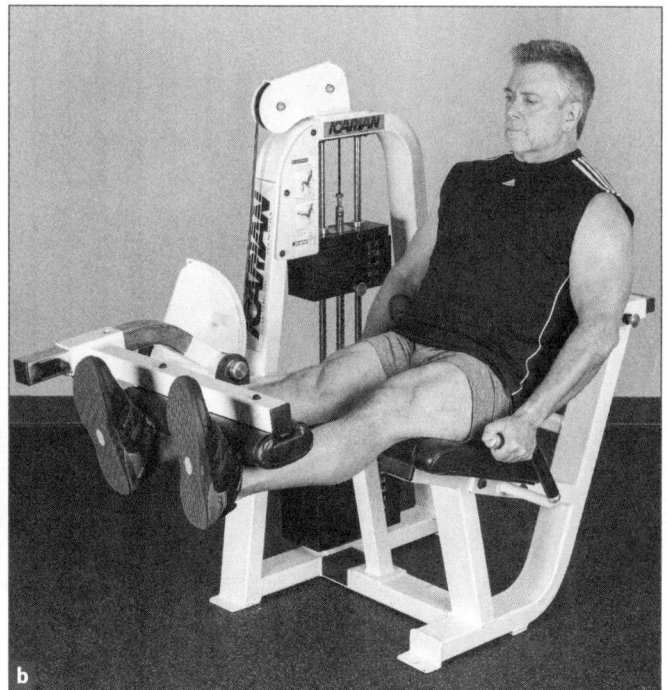

CHAD'S TAKE

To be honest, I prefer my older clientele to do squats, lunges, and step-ups because of the extra work on balance, coordination, and stabilization. None of that is required on the leg extension, but if you really want to connect to your quad muscles and feel the burn, this can't be beat.

CALF EXERCISES

I consider calf exercises optional for most clients. The truth is, unless you have very skinny calves that you're embarrassed by, you likely get enough calf work walking, hiking, and stair climbing. I've known countless men and women who didn't train calves in the gym at all, but through a combination of good calf genetics and an active lifestyle had calves even Arnold would be jealous of.

I will say that those with weak ankles who may have a history of rolling the ankle should probably do direct calf work to build up the muscles around it. Also, those prone to shin splints can benefit greatly from incorporating the anterior tibialis raise.

Machine Standing Calf Raise

The standing calf raise works the outer calf muscle, called the gastrocnemius, and also the deeper soleus muscle. The "gastroc" crosses the knee joint and needs the knee to be held straight to work effectively. The soleus does not cross the knee joint but can help extend the foot at the ankle in the straight leg position.

INSTRUCTION

- Stand with your feet a comfortable width apart. (I prefer to keep my feet together, but do what feels best for you.) Place the balls of your feet on the foot support with the rest of your foot off the platform. Lower your heels into a comfortable stretch and begin at the bottom of the movement (figure *a*).
- Drive up high on the balls of the feet, lifting your heels toward the ceiling (figure *b*).
- Lower your heels back to the starting position.

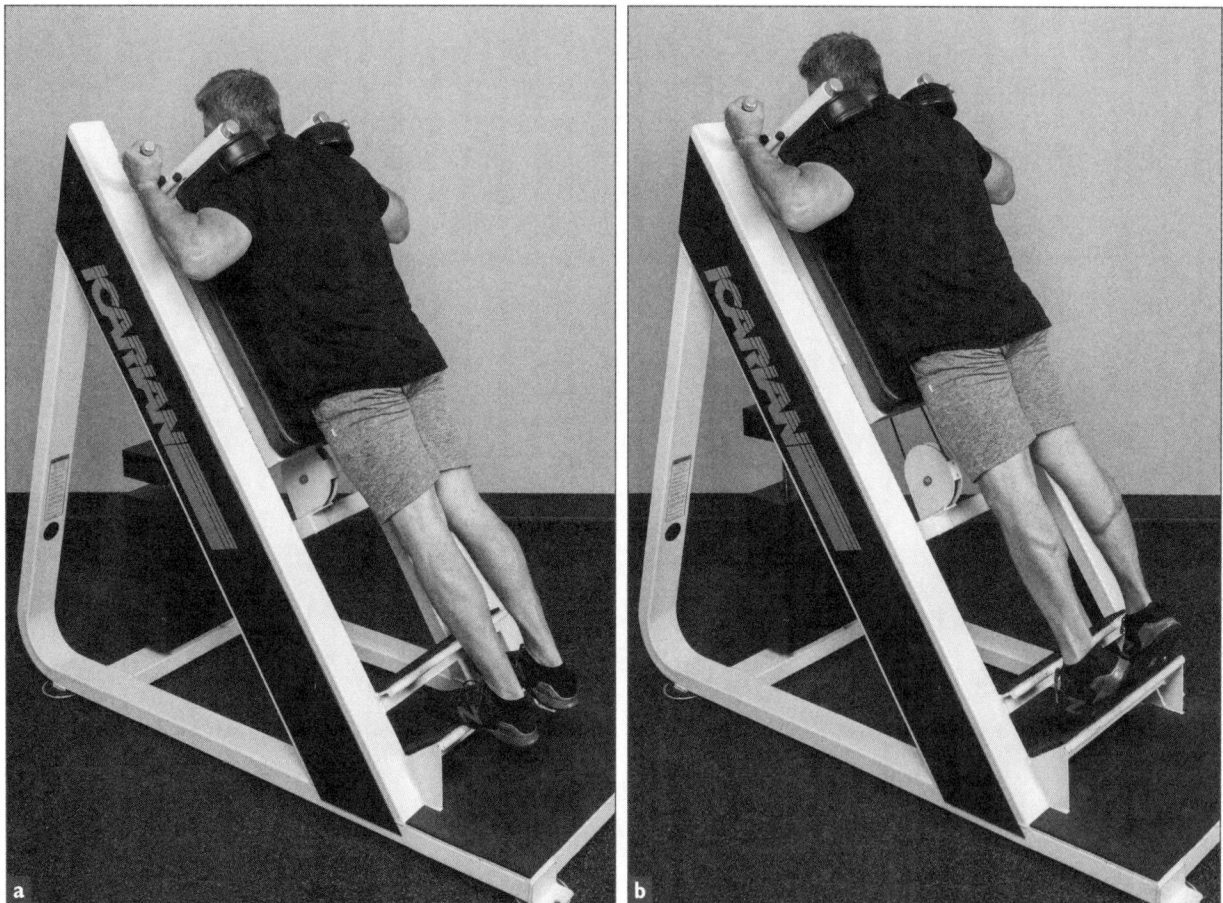

CHAD'S TAKE

If you're only going to do one exercise for calves, do standing calf raises, as both main muscles of the calves get stimulated. You can also play around with foot width (narrower or wider) and toe angle (in or out) and see what allows you to connect best to your calves and feels best on your feet and ankles.

Seated Calf Raise

This one targets the deeper soleus muscle, and because it's done with the knees bent, the gastroc cannot help the soleus. For this reason, many coaches prefer to just use the standing calf raise and consider the seated calf raise redundant. I still like the seated calf and incorporate it into my routines.

INSTRUCTION

- Sit on a seated calf raise machine with the balls of your feet on the foot plate and leg pad positioned on the thighs just above the knees. Raise the heels enough to disengage the safety arm, and lower the heels into the stretch position to begin the exercise (figure a).
- Drive through the balls of the feet to lift your heels up toward the ceiling (figure b).
- Lower your heels back to the starting position.

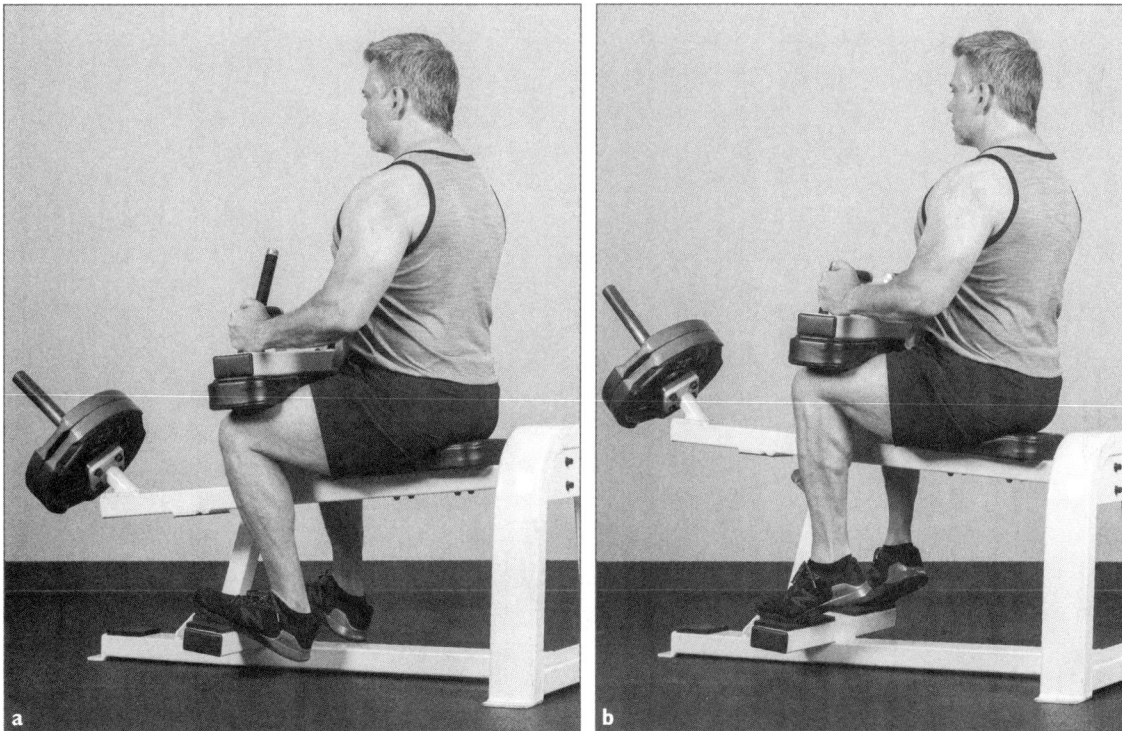

CHAD'S TAKE

If your gym has this machine, it's worth trying. Make sure you get a full stretch at the bottom, but don't get "bouncy" with the repetitions. I like to hold the stretch for two seconds each rep, which eliminates bouncing and adds a special burn to the exercise. Anyone with physique-competition aspirations should include this one for complete calf development.

Anterior Tibialis Raise

While I've seen some work-arounds, these are best done with a device called a dynamic axial resistance device (DARD). Most gyms likely won't have this, and you'll have to buy your own online. The DARD was the original brand, but search for "anterior tibialis bar" or "tib bar," and you'll be able to find one.

INSTRUCTION

- Place a DARD on top of both feet.
- If using the DARD on both feet, extend both legs on top of an exercise bench with the feet and weight hanging off the end and the toes pointed away from the body (figure *a*).
- Pull the toes up as far as possible while contracting the muscles on the front of the shin (figure *b*).
- Return to the start position.

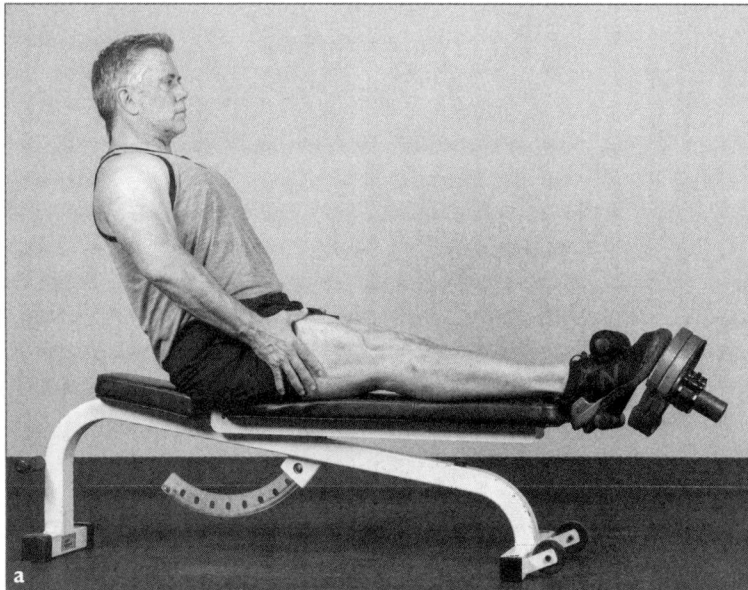

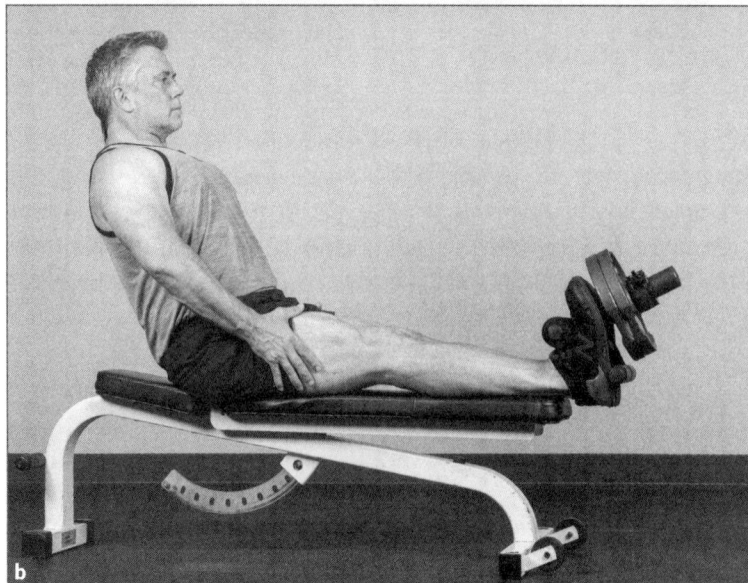

CHAD'S TAKE

I don't do this exercise very often, but I do have two DARDs at my gym in case I decide to use it with clients. Many active 50-somethings experience shin splints when exercising. If this is you, it is worth experimenting with anterior tibialis raises to strengthen those muscles. However, if you walk or hike on an incline often, your anterior tibialis may already be well developed, and you can skip these.

CHAPTER 10

Optimize Your Training

Remember recording songs off the radio with a dual-cassette boombox, fingers quivering above the REC/PAUSE button waiting for the perfect moment to cut in and out of the track, all while praying the DJ would please not chatter over the intro, then dubbing all those songs onto another tape in just the right order? Ah, a thing of beauty only Gen X can truly appreciate. Optimizing your training is like making the perfect mix tape.

Creating the optimal workout takes patience, tenacity, and a little bit of luck. First, we must remember that our pursuit of muscle and strength is not an "all or none" endeavor. Yet far too often, our training swings between too few (if any) workouts and too many (or too intense) workouts in an attempt to make up for missed training. We don't show up consistently enough to make real progress, then when we do finally hit the gym we train too hard, get super sore (or even injured), and end up missing even more workouts. Sound familiar?

Training programs should always consider the trainee's ability to stay consistent first and foremost. The program should be simple to follow and easy to repeat. Training sessions shouldn't be too long or too short, nor should they be too intense or too easy. They shouldn't cause injury, yet they need to be intense enough to stimulate a change in our physique. And they should allow us to make progress despite ongoing challenges with poor sleep habits, inadequate nutrition, and the various aches and pains found in an over-50 body.

The typical assumption is that if a little training is good, then more must be better. And while we do want progression and to achieve "more" (more weight, more reps, more work), we should start slowly and improve steadily. We need to coax our bodies to change, not try to beat them into submission. Overzealous trainees will try to add more weight *and* more reps *and* more sets *and* more workouts all at the same time, often leading to overtraining, burnout, and even injury. Obviously, that will kill your consistency.

Always be mindful of playing the long game when training after 50. This is a "rest of our lives" endeavor, not some short-term intervention, like the ones we've tried countless times before. Remember too that results must not only be earned but also maintained. And while hardcore quick-fix training and nutrition plans can be effective in the short term, they rarely produce a lifestyle you can stick with. So let's look at a number of ways to optimize your training week and get the most out of each individual training session and create your perfect workout mixtape.

FREQUENCY OF TRAINING

The first thing to consider when choosing a weight-training program is how many days per week you can commit to training. This is largely dictated by factors outside the gym—a hectic work and home schedule, for example. But it can also be influenced by your goals for strength training and your ability to recover from workouts.

Why are you strength training? Most recreational trainees 50 and older are focused on three things: losing body fat, toning up flabby muscles, and having more energy to get through the day and enjoy free time.

Some trainees may have a medical condition such as osteoporosis or diabetes, and their doctor has recommended strength training, so they're strictly interested in improving health outcomes. Still others may desire to push beyond general strength training and compete in masters level competitions such as powerlifting or bodybuilding or play sports like golf or tennis. The good news is that consistent training is the right prescription. We just need to tweak things a bit based on your goals.

I've broken up the programs in the chapters ahead based on the number of days per week you can commit to training. While many readers will simply be looking to get stronger and lose a little body fat, more advanced strategies are included in each programming chapter if you're looking to take things a bit further.

If you haven't been training regularly, I encourage you to start strength training twice weekly using the full-body workouts you'll find next in chapter 11. I've had scores of clients get strong and lean while weight training "just" two days a week. Two-day programs are especially suited for those who are physically active outside of weight training, be it yoga, Pilates, martial arts, or pickleball. Just remember that to continue to make progress in strength, you absolutely cannot miss workouts, except on rare occasions. One lifting day a week, while better than nothing, will slow progress to a glacial pace.

Most people will find three weightlifting days per week to be the sweet spot for maximizing results while still being able to recover from training and have the energy to pursue other physical endeavors on non-lifting days. You'll find my favorite three-day programs in chapter 12. Again, I prefer full-body routines on my three-day programs, but I do include some three-day split routines as well.

Some may do well with four weekly weight sessions, but these workouts will need to be brief and also split the areas of the body trained across multiple days. For those so inclined, check out my four-day programs in chapter 13. If you do decide to weight train four days per week, you will likely need to pay even more attention to your nutrition and sleep habits to ensure proper recovery from all these workouts. My recommendation is to focus on getting in two or three lifting sessions each week and using the other days to get in cardio or do things to promote recovery, such as massage.

EXERCISE SELECTION

You may be wondering how I decide what exercises to include in my programs. I take inspiration from this quote from Antoine de Saint-Exupéry: "Perfection is achieved, not when there is nothing left to add, but when there is nothing left to take away."

A brief aside: My wife (and one of my first clients!), Karen Baker Landers, a two-time Oscar-winning sound designer (*The Bourne Ultimatum*, *Skyfall*), turned me on to this quote because it inspires her choices when designing the sound-scape of a film. And while Saint-Exupéry was talking about airplane design, his premise is just as true for creating Oscar-winning sound design and developing smart weight-training programs. See the following sidebar for my tips on choosing exercises and other strategies for making the most of your training.

The programs in the next few chapters are guided by these principles. You will not see the type of two-hour marathon workouts we used to do in the '80s when we found our lifting programs in bodybuilding magazines, programs that were only appropriate for steroid-using high-level bodybuilders.

Chad's Tips to Maximize Program Results and Safety

• If a safer version of an exercise provides similar results, choose the safer option. I mentioned this in chapter 2, but I want to reiterate this point. Yes, all training has some risk involved, but we can minimize that risk by choosing exercises with a lesser chance of injury. If you're at a big commercial gym, you'll likely be able to use a machine version for most exercises. This is perfectly fine. You don't have to use the traditional barbell lifts such as the barbell back squat, the barbell bench press, or the straight bar deadlift. You can leg press or goblet squat, machine or dumbbell press, and kettlebell or hex bar deadlift. That's not to say barbells are bad. I'm 56 years old and still barbell bench press 300 pounds, but that works for me. Use exercises you feel safe with, and progress to more advanced ones as you feel more comfortable.

• Focus on exercises that work more muscles (big compound lifts) and do fewer isolation exercises for smaller muscles. You simply don't need five different biceps curl variations in a workout, no matter what you read in *Muscle & Fitness* in 1989.

• Do the minimum amount to see results. Ideally you will train in a range from the minimum effective dose to the maximum recoverable workload. I prefer you start lighter with fewer total sets and add volume (sets and reps) or intensity (weight) slowly.

• Work the entire body and leave no weak points. I prefer full-body workouts for this reason. Far too often men train chest and biceps only, and women focus solely on legs and glutes. This is a mistake, especially as we age. Weak points can lead to injury. We don't want a strong upper body and weak lower body or vice versa. Similarly, a strong chest but a weak back is a recipe for trouble.

TRAINING SESSION TIPS

In chapter 2 we covered overall principles of strength training and the specific principles of program design, but it's also important to consider strategies and techniques to optimize an individual training session.

The first question we must answer is "What are we trying to accomplish in this workout?" The answer should be straightforward, and 99 percent of the time it's "Provide enough stimulus to make my body bigger and stronger without injuring myself." But there will be those occasions where you are dealing with an injury or illness, or you are starting to feel run down and sore too often.

In these instances, the goal may be simply to lose as little ground as possible and "get the blood flowing and feel better leaving the gym than when you came in," and that's OK! Remember, consistency is key. I'd much rather have you do a light or abbreviated workout than no workout. But most workouts are about getting stronger, the progressive overload I mentioned in chapter 2.

Want to know the biggest secret to my success with both client results and my own training over the last four decades? No, it's not doing secret exercises or taking exotic supplements. And it's not "pedal to the metal" intensity during workouts or training every day. Quite simply, it's keeping a workout log.

I have actual physical logbooks filled with every weight, set, and rep performed in the gym by every client I've ever trained for more than 32 years, and I have over 40 years of my own training logs. In addition to the exercise data, I note any joint or muscle pain or discomfort, lack of sleep, a hangover, you name it. We don't only want to know what you did during the workout, but also indications of why you performed this way. The training data and notes will help inform what weight and how many reps to strive for the next time you do those exercises. For example, if you were getting over a cold the last time you performed an exercise, you may find you can easily push past the reps you did last time and even add weight. Conversely, if you are having a rough day, we may decide to go a bit lighter on the first set (or even all sets) and see how you do.

In the decade I trained clients at commercial gyms before opening my own studio, I noticed that I was often the only person in the gym logging their own workouts and was one of the only trainers keeping a log of their clients' workouts. (For a sample log sheet, see figure 10.1.) How can you expect to progress if you don't know what you did in the last workout and try to beat it the next time? That's the purpose of the journal and how I ensure both my clients and I achieve our goals.

Day:			Date:			Workout #:						
Warm-up/pre-workout cardio:						Post-workout cardio:						
		Set 1		Set 2		Set 3		Set 4		Set 5		
Body part	Exercise	Weight	Reps	Weight	Reps	Weight	Reps	Weight	Reps	Weight	Reps	Reps (sec.)
Notes and comments:												

FIGURE 10.1   Sample log sheet.

The following items should improve your workout log and help guide your training, no matter what your goal.

The Personal Record

Remember, the goal of each workout is to either lift a heavier weight than the last time you performed an exercise, or at least do more reps with the same weight as last time. Your goal should be to strive for a new personal record (PR) each workout. This gets harder to do the older we get and the longer we've been training, but improvement should still be the goal.

Typically, we think of a PR as the most weight you've ever lifted on an exercise for one repetition (your "one-repetition max" or 1RM). For example, my PR (1RM) on the bench press is 305 pounds. But I do not try to beat my 1RM each workout or even attempt a max that often.

The kind of PR I'm talking about is a cousin to the traditional 1RM PR. I simply want you to beat your performance from the previous time you performed an exercise. That might mean lifting 5 or 10 pounds heavier than the last workout or doing a rep or two more with the same weight. It might even be doing the same weight, sets, and reps but with better form.

For example, if the last time you did a machine chest press you did 3 sets of 10 reps with 50 pounds, next time try for 3 sets of 12 reps. Even if you "only" get sets of 12, 11, and 10 respectively, you still beat your total work by 3 reps. That's improvement. Then next time, try to beat the 12, 11, and 10 reps, and so on.

I generally recommend that most older trainees be able to do at least 8 repetitions with a weight but think 10- or 12-rep sets are more prudent because you'll need to use a slightly lighter weight, which tends to be easier on the joints. If you can't get at least 8 reps on all work sets, go lighter. Conversely, if you can easily do multiple sets of 15 reps in good form, go heavier next time. The only time I go fewer than 8 reps is when training a competitive powerlifter. Then we'll perform sets in the 1- to 5-rep range in addition to our regular higher rep work.

First Set Blues

This is something I coined years ago to describe the first heavy set of an exercise. There are times that no matter how thorough the warm-up, the first work set just feels kind of crummy. Still a bit stiff, maybe a little achy. Then the second set feels amazing, and clients often do more reps than their first set. But by set three, all bets are off. Maybe you can match set two, or maybe too much fatigue sets in.

Be aware that just because the first set feels out of sorts doesn't mean you need to go lighter or skip the exercise. As long as there were no sharp "stop" pains on the first set, see how the second set goes. You'll likely feel better and maybe get more reps than the first set.

However, if you start the second set and you have increased pain in a joint over the first set, stop immediately and either lighten the weight or skip the exercise and swap in something that doesn't cause pain. Doing a quick reset and adjusting joint angles might be all that is needed to make one of these "little pains" go away.

Rest Periods

Rest between sets is an important factor to consider and has been hotly debated. In general, we see better results (more reps with more weight, thus better strength and muscle gains) with longer rather than shorter rest periods.

Far too many trainees don't rest long enough between sets. This is a mistake. They are under the erroneous assumption that they should take as little rest as possible both between sets and between exercises during their strength sessions, because they mistakenly believe that the mark of an effective strength session is how out of breath and sweaty they are.

Traditionally, rest period recommendations have been 30 to 60 seconds if the goal is muscular endurance, 60 to 90 seconds if the goal is hypertrophy (size), and three to five minutes if the goal is strength. But many trainees desiring strength and hypertrophy end up using rest periods more applicable to endurance training. These short periods don't allow the muscular and nervous systems to rest long enough to perform optimally and promote size and strength gains.

Remember, the biggest reason we are doing resistance training in our 50s is to add as much muscle and strength as possible before we hit our 60s, when it gets even harder to fight Father Time. We need to use rest periods long enough to achieve these goals.

A study by Schoenfeld et al. (2016) showed that a longer rest period (three minutes) versus a shorter rest (60 seconds) was optimal for not only strength gains but also hypertrophy. Across various muscles studied, hypertrophy was about 7 percent greater with the longer rest period. Maximal strength increases on both the squat and bench press were similarly about 7 percent better when using a longer rest.

The authors speculate, based on their study and others referenced therein, that trainees should "at least" rest two minutes between sets. My experience over the last 30-plus years agrees with the research.

I know many of you who time your rest periods just won't be able to wait a full two minutes between sets, but please rest *at least* 90 seconds and preferably two to three minutes. Also, you don't have to use the same length rest period for each body part or exercise.

I do time my rests in my own training and note them in my workout journal. On smaller muscles like triceps, biceps, shoulders, and calves, I find I'm recovered and ready after a two-minute rest. For the bigger muscles like the back, chest, and thighs, I take a two-minute rest after warm-up sets and three minutes after work sets. For my super-heavy, low-rep (1 to 5) bench press sets, I find I need at least four minutes between sets.

However, if it feels too tedious to time your rest periods and is an impediment to training, you don't have to do it. In that instance, I recommend resting as long as you need in order to work hard again on the next set. The worst thing that will happen if you don't rest long enough is you'll get far fewer reps on the next set. Just don't rest so long that you cool down or make your workouts any longer than they need to be.

If you are fairly in tune with your body, you'll probably know when you're ready to perform another set. Just be aware that if you have a significant drop-off in number of reps from set to set, you likely aren't resting long enough. For example, if you complete 12 reps on the first set but can only do 6 or 7 on the second set, you didn't rest long enough. Aim for no more than a drop-off of 1 to 3 reps between sets.

Rep Speed or "Tempo"

How fast should you perform each repetition? First, I think it's overkill to try to time each rep in your head. You'll often find programs with a recommended tempo of something like 2/0/2 to 4/2/2 or similar. These numbers denote the number of seconds to lower the weight (the eccentric phase), how long to pause between phases, and how quickly to lift the weight (the concentric phase).

I find most people have a hard enough time concentrating on what rep they are on while also concentrating on proper form. Imagine counting in your head "One, two, three, four (negative), one, two (pause), one, two (concentric) and *one*" (rep). Now keep doing that for each rep of each set! Tedious and confusing.

That does *not* mean to mimic a "gym fails" video online and perform reps as fast as possible with no control. Nor does it mean you should go "super slow." I've seen recommendations to take as long as 45 seconds to complete one repetition! While hard to do, this is not at all necessary and is actually not optimal for building muscle (Schoenfeld, Ogborn, and Krieger 2015).

My advice is to keep it simple. You should be able to lower a weight under control and then lift it as quickly as possible while still controlling the weight. I always say, "Control the weight, don't let the weight control you." I don't typically have clients pause between the eccentric and concentric phases, but a short pause of one or two seconds will dissipate any momentum and the "stretch reflex."

You will be able to lift heavier if you use this stretch reflex to your advantage by not pausing. But I find a short pause to eliminate this is good for people who have poor control and tend to "bounce" out of the bottom. And for older lifters, I think the slight pause lessens the chance of injury by the need to use a bit lighter weight and lessens the chance of overstretching the joint in the negative.

But again, don't overthink this. Controlled eccentric, quick pause (if any), fast but controlled concentric.

WRAPPING UP

Remember, training to build muscle and strength is fairly simple and straightforward. Show up to the gym consistently. Endeavor to do more "work" than the last time, either by lifting more weight or doing more total reps than before. Keep a journal to log your workout and any information that may have impacted your performance.

Control the speed of your reps and be sure to take enough rest between sets and exercises to allow you to give your best effort to achieve a new PR on as many exercises as you can. And always remember, your results will be as good as your consistent efforts. Commit to strength training two to four times each week and make your goals a reality.

Now that you know what makes a great workout mixtape, let's dive into the next three chapters and check out the program mixtapes I've already made for you and decide which one you should listen to first.

CHAPTER 11

Two-Days-a-Week Programs

A mixtape is the perfect analogy for my two-day programs. We'll do side A on day 1, flip the tape, and do side B on day 2. Even if you decide to jump into a three-day or even four-day program, start with the two assessment workouts described in this chapter.

As I mentioned in chapter 4, I don't do traditional strength testing or assessments because I consider each workout to be an ongoing assessment. Thus, my initial workout with clients is composed of exercises I feel give a good evaluation of the basic movement patterns while also providing the client with a good example of what training with me is like. The assessment continues on the second training session using other exercises that round out the basic movement patterns. These workouts are typically not very strenuous and should feel easy. That doesn't mean clients don't feel tired afterward or can't get sore from the workouts, but that's not my goal.

I do these workouts with every new client, no matter how old they are or how long they've been training or how many days per week they will ultimately be training with me. I need to see how their body works and check their current level of mastery of technique on these exercises, and I will, of course, correct their form when appropriate. I don't want the first few workouts to be overwhelming. I want them to knock the rust off if it's been a while since they've trained and provide a positive launching point for the inevitably harder workouts to come.

I check the following movement patterns:

Upper-body push (horizontal, vertical)

Upper-body pull (horizontal, vertical)

Lower body (quad dominant, hip dominant)

Core (antiflexion, antirotation)

Note: I intentionally leave out exercises for the smaller muscles—biceps, triceps, and calves—to save time because these initial workouts take longer with the added teaching time.

I usually use the following exercises for the first two workouts:

Day One

Step-up (quad-dominant lower body)

Push-up (rack) (horizontal push)

Machine seated row (horizontal pull)

Dead bug (antiflexion)

Day Two

Pull-up (assisted) or machine pull-down (vertical pull)

Seated dumbbell shoulder press (or landmine press) (vertical push)

Hip thrust (hip-dominant lower body)

Pallof press (antirotation)

I chose these exercises because they are a good starting point for most people. For example, a push-up in the rack (where I can adjust starting height and use a closed-chain movement) is doable for most people and has less risk of injury than a barbell or dumbbell bench press. Also, although I usually include assisted pull-ups during the second or third workout, certain clients may not be strong enough to do them even with the assistance of the entire weight stack. So, I will instead use a different vertical pull (likely a machine pull-down). Also, if you are unable to do unassisted pull-ups and your gym doesn't have an assisted pull-up machine, you'll need to use a cable or machine pull-down instead.

The same holds true for step-ups. Nearly every one of my clients has been able to start with a 12-inch box, but some needed a 9-inch or even 6-inch box, and some simply didn't have the strength (or balance or coordination) to do them at all, and instead started with a more stable, bilateral exercise such as a sit-to-stand or box squat.

Note the overhead pressing exercise on day two. The one assessment I do before overhead pressing is the shoulder flexion test. If someone passes the test, I will start them with seated dumbbell shoulder presses. If not, we'll start with the landmine and work on improving shoulder flexion before using dumbbells overhead.

THE BARE MINIMUM

This program takes my assessment workouts and just keeps rolling. It is for those who have never really trained before, have had a long layoff since strength training, or who simply want to be in the gym as briefly as possible. The brevity of these workouts makes this program a great beginning routine for those individuals who are naturally thin and have a hard time adding muscle or recovering from workouts. The bare minimum program is a minimalist full-body workout designed to be done two days a week, with workout A done on day one and workout B on day two. Repeat the program for four to eight weeks or as long as you continue to make progress.

TABLE 11.1   Bare Minimum Two-Days-a-Week Program

Workout A			
Movement focus	**Exercise**	**Sets and reps**	**Page #**
Horizontal pull	Machine seated row	3 × 10-15	68
Horizontal push	Dumbbell bench press	3 × 10-15	51
Quad-dominant lower body	Goblet squat	3 × 10-15	134
Core	Dead bug	3 × 10-15 per side	122

Workout B			
Movement focus	**Exercise**	**Sets and reps**	**Page #**
Vertical pull	Lat pull-down	3 × 10-15	71
Vertical push	Seated dumbbell shoulder press	3 × 10-15	85
Hip-dominant lower body	Hip thrust	3 × 10-15	145
Core	Pallof press	2-3 × 30 sec per side	120

THE BARE MINIMUM PLUS CARDIO INTERVALS

This program is for those who don't have the time to do cardio on nonlifting days but desire to get some cardiovascular conditioning in while also doing the bare minimum amount of strength training. It is not ideal for those who have trouble gaining muscle and recovering from workouts but is a great way to be able to lift heavy and get a bit of cardio in (in contrast to circuit training, which is more conditioning using weights than true strength training combined with intervals). After two to four weeks, trainees can decide to continue with this program for another four weeks or progress to my go-to program.

TABLE 11.2   Bare Minimum Plus Cardio Intervals Two-Days-a-Week Program

Workout A			
Movement focus	**Exercise**	**Sets and reps or time**	**Page #**
Horizontal pull	Machine seated row	3 × 10-15	68
Cardio interval	Elliptical	2 min	n/a
Horizontal push	Dumbbell bench press	3 × 10-15	51
Cardio interval	Elliptical	2 min	n/a
Quad-dominant lower body	Goblet squat	3 × 10-15	134
Cardio interval	Elliptical	2 min	n/a
Core	Dead bug	3 × 10-15 per side	122

(continued)

Table 11.2 Bare Minimum Plus Cardio Intervals Two-Days-a-Week Program *(continued)*

	Workout B		
Movement focus	**Exercise**	**Sets and reps or time**	**Page #**
Vertical pull	Pull-up	3 × 10-15	72
Cardio interval	Recumbent bike	2 min	n/a
Vertical push	Seated dumbbell shoulder press	3 × 10-15	85
Cardio interval	Recumbent bike	2 min	n/a
Hip-dominant lower body	Hip thrust	3 × 10-15	145
Cardio interval	Recumbent bike	2 min	n/a
Core	Pallof press	2-3 × 30 sec per side	120

THE GT PROGRAM

My "go-to" program (GT) is for the average person looking to get stronger and leaner and fitter. Although it's listed as an 8- to 12-week program, you could literally run this program for months if not years (which I've done with scores of clients).

One caveat if you're going to run this program year-round: I highly recommend experimenting with other exercises for the different movement patterns. While there's no such thing as muscle confusion, it's still a good idea to prevent boredom and possible repetitive stress by varying the exercises you choose.

Note the two main differences between the bare minimum and the GT programs:

1. The GT adds direct work for the arms and calves.
2. The GT includes an additional C workout for more variety.

In week one, you'll do workout A on day one and workout B on day two. In week two, you'll do workout C on day one and workout A on day two. In week three, you'll do workout B on day one and workout C on day two. Repeat the sequence for as many weeks as desired.

TABLE 11.3 GT Two-Days-a-Week Program

	Workout A		
Movement focus	**Exercise**	**Sets and reps**	**Page #**
Horizontal pull	Machine seated row	3 × 10-15	68
Horizontal push	Dumbbell bench press	3 × 10-15	51
Quad-dominant lower body	Goblet squat	3 × 10-15	134
Triceps	Cable triceps push-down	3 × 10-15	111
Core (sagittal plane)	Dead bug	3 × 10-15 per side	122

Workout B			
Movement focus	**Exercise**	**Sets and reps**	**Page #**
Vertical pull	Pull-up	3 × 10-15	72
Vertical push	Seated dumbbell shoulder press	3 × 10-15	85
Hip-dominant lower body	Hip thrust	3 × 10-15	144
Biceps	Dumbbell hammer curl	3 × 10-15	99
Core (transverse plane)	Pallof press	2-3 × 30 sec per side	120

Workout C			
Movement focus	**Exercise**	**Sets and reps**	**Page #**
Mid-range pull	Face pull	3 × 10-15	77
Incline push	Incline dumbbell bench press	3 × 10-15	61
Combo lower body	Reverse lunge	3 × 10-15	141
Delts or calves	Machine standing calf raise	3 × 10-15	156
Core (frontal plane or combo)	Stir the pot	3 × 10-15 each direction	119

THE GT WITH INTERVALS

The GT with intervals program is the main program I use to get actors and musicians in shape, although we usually use the three-day-a-week version. It's a great overall program to get strong, lean, and fit.

There are two options for doing intervals with the longer GT workouts. Option one features four intervals total, and option two has two intervals. Note: You could leave out the final interval on option one if you wanted to do only three intervals.

TABLE 11.4   GT With Intervals Two-Days-a-Week Program

Workout A			
Movement focus	**Exercise**	**Sets and reps or time**	**Page #**
Horizontal pull	Machine seated row	3 × 10-15	68
Cardio interval (1)	Recumbent bike	2 min	n/a
Horizontal push	Dumbbell bench press	3 × 10-15	51
Cardio interval (1, 2)	Recumbent bike	2 min	n/a
Quad-dominant lower body	Goblet squat	3 × 10-15	134
Cardio interval (1)	Recumbent bike	2 min	n/a
Triceps	Cable triceps push-down	3 × 10-15	111
Cardio interval (1, 2)	Recumbent bike	2 min	n/a
Core (sagittal plane)	Dead bug	3 × 10-15 per side	122

(continued)

Table 11.4   GT With Intervals Two-Days-a-Week Program *(continued)*

Workout B			
Movement focus	**Exercise**	**Sets and reps or time**	**Page #**
Vertical pull	Pull-up	3 × 10-15	72
Cardio interval (1)	Fan bike	2 min	n/a
Vertical push	Seated dumbbell shoulder press	3 × 10-15	85
Cardio interval (1, 2)	Fan bike	2 min	n/a
Hip-dominant lower body	Hip thrust	3 × 10-15	145
Cardio interval (1)	Fan bike	2 min	n/a
Biceps	Dumbbell hammer curl	3 × 10-15	97
Cardio interval (1, 2)	Fan bike	2 min	n/a
Core (transverse plane)	Pallof press	2-3 × 30 sec per side	120

Workout C			
Movement focus	**Exercise**	**Sets and reps or time**	**Page #**
Mid-range pull	Face pull	3 × 10-15	77
Cardio interval (1)	Stepping machine	2 min	n/a
Incline push	Incline dumbbell bench press	3 × 10-15	61
Cardio interval (1, 2)	Stepping machine	2 min	n/a
Combo lower body	Reverse lunge	3 × 10-15	141
Cardio interval (1)	Stepping machine	2 min	n/a
Delts or calves	Machine standing calf raise	3 × 10-15	156
Cardio interval (1, 2)	Stepping machine	2 min	n/a
Core (frontal plane or combo)	Stir the pot	3 × 10-15 each direction	119

I wouldn't recommend the GT with intervals programs for those who like to do high-intensity interval training on their off days from lifting. Too many high-intensity intervals too often in addition to intense resistance training is a recipe for burnout, fatigue, and possible injury.

It's likely OK to include intervals in your program if you're only doing zone two cardio on off days but no high-intensity intervals. You'll have to determine that for yourself based on your recovery ability. Consult chapter 14 for an in-depth look at cardio and recovery.

CHAPTER 12

Three-Days-a-Week Programs

Think of my three-day programs like the original Star Wars trilogy. Day 1 is *A New Hope*, day 2 is *The Empire Strikes Back*, day 3 is *Return of the Jedi*. It doesn't get any better than this. And while each film is great alone, and regardless of which one is your favorite (it's gotta be *Empire*, right?), when they are combined and done in order, it's perfection. I think most people will see their best results knocking out their own trilogy each week at the gym, and it's why I recommend three-day programs most to my clients.

My three-day programs take the essence of my two-day programs but complete all three workouts (ABC) in the same week. This means that instead of taking three weeks to repeat each workout twice, it will take only two weeks to do so. As you might imagine, doing the same amount of work in a third less time should lead to quicker results.

For those who don't do other exercise activities regularly outside of strength training, I recommend three-day programs. For those regularly committed to other activities outside of the gym (e.g., pickleball, golf, Pilates, yoga), try the two-day programs in chapter 11 first, and add a third day only if you are recovering well from all your activities.

THREE-DAY GT

The three-day go-to is my gold standard for three-day programs. It allows for heavy weights across a variety of exercises and planes of motion in a relatively short workout (40 to 60 minutes). Like my two-day GT, you can roll with this program for years. Simply vary the exercises to prevent boredom. Perform workout A on day one, workout B on day two, and workout C on day three of your training week. Repeat the sequence for as many weeks as desired.

TABLE 12.1   GT Three-Days-a-Week Program

Workout A			
Movement focus	**Exercise**	**Sets and reps**	**Page #**
Horizontal pull	Pendlay row	3 × 10-15	67
Horizontal push	Machine chest press	3 × 10-15	54
Quad-dominant lower body	Leg press	3 × 10-15	136
Triceps	Dumbbell skull crusher	3 × 10-15	110
Core (sagittal plane)	Hanging ab raise	3 × 10-15	130
Workout B			
Movement focus	**Exercise**	**Sets and reps**	**Page #**
Vertical pull	Lat pull-down	3 × 10-15	71
Vertical push	Single-arm landmine press	3 × 10-15 per side	94
Hip-dominant lower body	Hex bar deadlift	3 × 10-15	138
Biceps	Cable EZ curl	3 × 10-15	101
Core (transverse plane)	Pallof hold	2-3 × 30 sec per side	n/a
Workout C			
Movement focus	**Exercise**	**Sets and reps**	**Page #**
Mid-range pull	Single-arm dumbbell row on bench	3 × 10-15 per side	75
Incline push	Incline barbell bench press	3 × 10-15	62
Combo lower body	Step-up	3 × 10-15 per side	143
Delts or calves	Seated calf raise	3 × 10-15	157
Core (frontal plane or combo)	Farmer walk	3 × 30-60 sec each side	121

THREE-DAY GT WITH INTERVALS

The addition of intervals to the three-day GT makes for a longer, more fatiguing workout but is ideal for those who simply won't do cardio on non-weight-training days. This is the workout I've used with my celebrity clients for over two decades. Again, there are two options for including intervals based on your personal preferences, adding either four intervals (option one) or two intervals (option two). If you want to, you can leave out the last interval in option one to have only three intervals.

TABLE 12.2   GT With Intervals Three-Days-a-Week Program

Workout A			
Movement focus	**Exercise**	**Sets and reps or time**	**Page #**
Horizontal pull	Two-dumbbell chest-supported row	3 × 10-15	70
Cardio interval (1)	Recumbent bike	2 min	n/a

Workout A (continued)			
Movement focus	**Exercise**	**Sets and reps or time**	**Page #**
Horizontal push	Barbell bench press	3 × 10-15	52
Cardio interval (1, 2)	Recumbent bike	2 min	n/a
Quad-dominant lower body	Bulgarian split squat	3 × 10-15	135
Cardio interval (1)	Recumbent bike	2 min	n/a
Triceps	Cable overhead triceps extension	3 × 10-15	114
Cardio interval (1, 2)	Recumbent bike	2 min	n/a
Core (sagittal plane)	Plank	2 × 30-60 sec	125
Workout B			
Movement focus	**Exercise**	**Sets and reps or time**	**Page #**
Vertical pull	Pull-up	3 × 10-15	72
Cardio interval (1)	Fan bike	2 min	n/a
Vertical push	Seated dumbbell shoulder press	3 × 10-15	85
Cardio interval (1, 2)	Fan bike	2 min	n/a
Hip-dominant lower body	Romanian deadlift	3 × 10-15	152
Cardio interval (1)	Fan bike	2 min	n/a
Biceps	Dumbbell spider curl	3 × 10-15	104
Cardio interval (1, 2)	Fan bike	2 min	n/a
Core (transverse plane)	Pallof hold	2-3 × 30 sec per side	n/a
Workout C			
Movement focus	**Exercise**	**Sets and reps or time**	**Page #**
Mid-range pull	Inverted row	3 × 10-15	76
Cardio interval (1)	Stepping machine	2 min	n/a
Incline push	Incline dumbbell bench press	3 × 10-15	61
Cardio interval (1, 2)	Stepping machine	2 min	n/a
Combo lower body	Walking lunge	3 × 10-15	n/a
Cardio interval (1)	Stepping machine	2 min	n/a
Delts or calves	Single-arm cable lateral raise	3 × 10-15 per side	88
Cardio interval (1, 2)	Stepping machine	2 min	n/a
Core (frontal plane or combo)	Body saw	3 × 10-15 each direction	126

PUSH–PULL–LEGS PROGRAM

This program is more for bodybuilding enthusiasts who have only three days to train each week. It has two upper-body days (one push, one pull) and one lower-body day. I don't recommend this program for the average person because each body part is being trained only one day per week. As such, these workouts tend to be longer and harder on the areas they are working. I prefer slightly less intensity but more frequency with my general population clients.

TABLE 12.3   Push–Pull–Legs Three-Days-a-Week Program

Workout A			
Push	**Exercise**	**Sets and reps**	**Page #**
Horizontal push	Dumbbell bench press	3 × 10-15	51
Vertical push	Seated dumbbell shoulder press	3 × 10-15	85
Incline push	Incline dumbbell bench press	3 × 10-15	61
Lateral delt	Single-arm cable lateral raise	2-3 × 10-15 per side	88
Triceps	Cable triceps pushdown	2-3 × 10-15	111
Core (sagittal plane)	Dead bug	3 × 10-15 per side	122
Workout B			
Pull	**Exercise**	**Sets and reps**	**Page #**
Horizontal pull	Machine seated row	3 × 10-15	68
Vertical pull	Pull-up or lat pull-down	3 × 10-15	72, 71
Mid-range pull	Face pull	2-3 × 10-15	77
Rear delt/external rotation	Cable external rotation	2-3 × 10-15	82
Biceps	Dumbbell hammer curl	2-3 × 10-15	97
Core (transverse plane)	Pallof press	2-3 × 30 sec per side	120
Workout C			
Legs	**Exercise**	**Sets and reps**	**Page #**
Hip-dominant lower body	Goblet squat	3 × 10-15	134
Quad-dominant lower body	Reverse lunge	3 × 10-15	141
Hamstring specific	Seated leg curl	3 × 10-15	150
Glute specific	Hip thrust	3 × 10-15	145
Calves	Machine standing calf raise	3 × 10-15	157
Core (frontal plane or combo)	Stir the pot	3 × 10-15 each direction	119

CHAPTER 13

Four-Days-a-Week Programs

The four-day programs are the training equivalent of The A-Team. Hannibal, Face, B.A., and Murdock are four specialists with one mission. Perhaps unsurprisingly, I typically reserve four-day programs for celebrity clients who need to get in shape fast or highly motivated clients who don't do other physical activities outside the gym. I've found that most clients over 50 with busy schedules can neither be consistent with four-day programs nor recover fully between workouts once adding a fourth day of lifting. However, I did include a few four-day programs for those who have the desire and recovery ability to thrive on them. If your sleep and nutrition are dialed in, you can make incredible progress on a four-day schedule.

While most people can do my two- and three-day go-to (GT) programs for months (or even years), the same may not be true for four-day programs. Save them for times of year when you can commit to better sleep, great nutrition, and less life stress. Maybe for four to six weeks in a row. Then go back to a two- or three-day program.

The biggest difference in my four-day programs is that they exclusively use a body part split; no full-body sessions here, so like The A-Team, you'll need each one to show up to complete your mission. Also, I do not recommend concurrent training using cardio intervals on four-day programs like those in my two- and three-day programs. That's like calling on The A-Team and the Ninja Turtles—too much going on there. For cardio options on non-weight-training days, check out chapter 14.

FOUR-DAY GT

As mentioned, the four-day GT programs use a body part split instead of full-body routines. These programs are suitable for both general strength and bodybuilding. Here are two different splits to try:

1. **Push/pull split** (table 13.1): This program is different than the push–pull–legs three-day split because each workout includes both upper- and low-

er-body exercises, putting quad-dominant exercises and calves on push days and hip-dominant exercises, hamstrings, and glutes on pull days.

2. **Upper/lower split** (table 13.2): As the name suggests, this program divides the work into upper- and lower-body days. This allows for more exercises to target those areas during the training session.

TABLE 13.1 Push/Pull Split Four-Days-a-Week Program

Push 1			
Movement focus	**Exercise**	**Sets and reps**	**Page #**
Horizontal push	Dumbbell bench press	3 × 10-15	51
Vertical push	Seated dumbbell shoulder press	3 × 10-15	85
Quad-dominant lower body	Goblet squat	3 × 10-15	134
Calves	Machine standing calf raise	2-3 × 12-20	156
Triceps	Cable triceps pushdown	2-3 × 10-15	111
Core (sagittal plane)	Dead bug	3 × 10-15 each side	122

Pull 1			
Movement focus	**Exercise**	**Sets and reps**	**Page #**
Horizontal pull	Machine seated row	3 × 10-15	68
Vertical pull	Pull-up or lat pull-down	3 × 10-15	72, 71
Hamstring specific	Seated leg curl	3 × 10-15	150
Rear delts, external rotation	Face pull or cable external rotation	2-3 × 10-15	77, 82
Biceps	Dumbbell hammer curl	2-3 × 10-15	97
Core (transverse plane)	Pallof press	2-3 × 30 sec each side	120

Push 2			
Movement focus	**Exercise**	**Sets and reps**	**Page #**
Incline push	Incline dumbbell bench press or machine chest press	3 × 10-15	61, 54
Lateral delt	Single-arm cable lateral raise	2-3 × 10-15 each side	88
Quad specific or combo	Reverse lunge	3 × 10-15 each side	141
Calves	Seated calf raise	3 × 10-15	157
Triceps	Cable overhead triceps extension	2-3 × 10-15	114
Core (frontal plane)	Farmer walk	2-3 × 30-60 sec each side	121

Pull 2			
Movement focus	**Exercise**	**Sets and reps**	**Page #**
Hip-dominant lower body	Hex bar deadlift	3 × 10-15	138
Mid-range pull	Face pull	2-3 × 10-15	77
Glute specific	Hip thrust	3 × 10-15	145
Rear delts, external rotation	Cable external rotation	2-3 × 10-15	82
Biceps	Cable EZ curl	2-3 × 10-15	101
Core (combo)	Stir the pot	3 × 10-15 each direction	119

TABLE 13.2   Upper/Lower Split Four-Days-a-Week Program

Upper A			
Movement focus	**Exercise**	**Sets and reps**	**Page #**
Vertical pull	Pull-up or lat pull-down	3 × 10-15	72, 71
Vertical push	Seated dumbbell shoulder press	3 × 10-15	85
Lateral delt	Single-arm cable lateral raise	2-3 × 10-15 each side	88
Triceps	Cable triceps pushdown	2-3 × 10-15	111
Core (sagittal plane)	Dead bug	3 × 10-15	122
Lower A			
Movement focus	**Exercise**	**Sets and reps**	**Page #**
Quad-dominant lower body	Goblet squat	3 × 10-15	134
Hamstring specific	Seated leg curl	3 × 10-15	150
Glute specific or combo	Hip thrust	3 × 10-15	145
Calves	Machine standing calf raise	3 × 10-15	156
Core (transverse plane)	Pallof press	2-3 × 30 sec each side	120
Upper B			
Movement focus	**Exercise**	**Sets and reps**	**Page #**
Horizontal pull	Machine seated row	3 × 10-15	68
Horizontal or incline push	Flat or incline dumbbell bench press	3 × 10-15	51, 61
Rear delt, external rotation	Face pull or cable external rotation	2-3 × 10-15	77, 82
Biceps	Dumbbell hammer curl	2-3 × 10-15	97
Core (frontal plane)	Farmer walk	2-3 × 30-60 sec each side	121

(continued)

Table 13.2 *(continued)*

Lower B			
Movement focus	**Exercise**	**Sets and reps**	**Page #**
Hip-dominant lower body	Hex bar deadlift	3 × 8-12	138
Quad specific	Leg extension machine	3 × 10-15	154
Glute specific or combo	Reverse lunge	3 × 10-15	141
Calves	Seated calf raise	3 × 10-15	157
Core (combo)	Stir the pot	3 × 10-15 each direction	119

CHAPTER 14

Cardio and Recovery

I almost named this chapter "Everything I Know About Recovery I Learned from Dungeons & Dragons." Because let's be honest, any Gen Xer who spent their youth rolling d20s knows you don't just charge into your next encounter without a long rest to restore your hit points. Now that we're on the other side of 50, it's more important than ever to support our strength-training goals with smart recovery and solid cardio. In addition to the nutrition strategies we covered in chapter 3, it's time we examine the other parts of the equation: building cardiorespiratory fitness and mastering the art of recovery. This is how we keep showing up at full strength, ready for battle, whatever the next roll of the dice brings.

In the introduction I mentioned how for decades older adults were urged to focus their fitness endeavors on cardio and eschew weight training. Even young athletes were once told they had to make a choice—cardio *or* weights. Advocates of each training modality thought the other type of exercise would be detrimental: weightlifting would make you stiff, bulky, and slow; and any cardio would kill your muscle and strength gains.

We now know that regardless of age or training goals, we shouldn't choose between cardio *or* weights but instead should combine both cardio *and* weights. However, we do need to make sure our cardio workouts are appropriate for our goals of building muscle and strength after 50. As such, my advice for cardio workouts keeps those goals in mind . . . this is not a book to improve your ultra-marathon time.

But remember, even the perfect combination of strength training and cardio workouts won't yield the desired results if you are unable to recover from these workouts. Recovery can be challenging at any age, but especially so north of 50. So, let's dig into some simple cardio and recovery advice to maximize your strength-training results.

CARDIO

When actor William "Billy" Zabka called me to train him to reprise his *Karate Kid* character, Johnny Lawrence, for *Cobra Kai*, we didn't have a lot of time to get ready. Plus it had been 35 years since Johnny/Billy "swept the leg" and Billy was now in his '50s, so we needed the right combination of both cardio and weights to get him ready.

The combination of strength and cardiovascular conditioning forms the bedrock of any well-rounded fitness regimen, offering many benefits that extend far beyond the weight room. First, aerobic fitness plays a pivotal role in supporting overall cardiovascular health. Regular aerobic exercise has been shown to improve heart health by strengthening the heart muscle, lowering blood pressure, and increasing HDL (good) cholesterol levels, thus reducing the risk of heart disease and stroke (American Heart Association 2023).

Cardio has also been shown to enhance respiratory function, increase lung capacity, and improve oxygen delivery to working muscles, thereby enhancing endurance and delaying the onset of fatigue during strength-training sessions (Oja et al. 2011). Yes, this means you can train harder, longer.

While strength training is renowned for its ability to build lean muscle mass and boost metabolism, the addition of cardio helps accelerate the rate of calorie expenditure, facilitating fat loss and promoting a leaner, more defined physique (Willis et al. 2012).

Another compelling argument for incorporating cardio into your strength-training regimen lies in its profound impact on overall well-being. Regular aerobic exercise has been shown to reduce symptoms of anxiety and depression, enhance mood, and improve cognitive function, thus promoting mental clarity and emotional resilience (Mandolesi et al. 2018). All important for those over 50.

And if you still need convincing to do your cardio, remember this: cardiorespiratory fitness…as measured by $\dot{V}O_2$ max…is one of the single best predictors of how long you'll live. In a 122,000-person Cleveland Clinic study, each 1-MET (approximately $3.5 \text{ ml} \cdot \text{kg}^{-1} \cdot \text{min}^{-1}$) bump in VO_2 max cut all-cause mortality by about 10 percent, and "elite" performers enjoyed an 80 percent lower risk of death than the least-fit group (Mandsager et al. 2018). Similar results from the 750,000-participant Veterans Exercise Testing Study showed a four-fold survival advantage for those at the highest fitness levels, with no evidence of an "upper ceiling" where extra fitness stops helping, in fact, benefits persisted well into the seventies and beyond (Kokkinos et al. 2022) Translation for the Gen-X adventurer: boosting your $\dot{V}O_2$ max is like equipping a +3 Amulet of Constitution, padding your hit-point pool with a few extra decades for the long-haul campaign…no chrono-shift spell required.

So, how exactly should one integrate cardio into their strength-training routine? The key lies in striking a balance between the two modalities, so they complement and enhance each other, just like rolling a well-rounded character in Dungeons & Dragons. You wouldn't dump all your points into strength and neglect dexterity or constitution, and the same goes for your training. This might involve dedicating specific days to cardiovascular workouts like running, cycling, or swimming or incorporating shorter bouts of high-intensity interval training (HIIT) to keep your fitness stats well-balanced.

Alternatively, you might opt for concurrent training, where cardio and strength exercises are performed in the same workout session. This approach allows for maximal efficiency and time savings, while still reaping the benefits of both modalities (Kraemer and Ratamess 2004), and it's what I do with most of my celebrity clients who need to get lean quickly. Look back on chapters 11 and 12, where I included options for concurrent training with intervals on my two- and three-day programs.

Although I use concurrent training liberally with clients, I personally don't usually do structured concurrent training, although I have been known to attempt a PR on a sprint distance on the Concept 2 rowing ergometer after my weight-lifting workout. Instead I like to include cardio on my non-weight-training days. This comes in the form of one of two options: Zone 2 training and HIIT training.

Zone 2 training refers to the percentage of your maximum heart rate you maintain during training based on five heart rate zones (figure 14.1).

Common recommendations for Zone 2 training are 120 minutes a week for beginners and 180 to 240 minutes weekly for more advanced trainees. This much cardio is only possible because the intensity of Zone 2 is so low, and it's very easy to recover from. However, I don't do anywhere near this much, and I don't think most 50-somethings who aren't early retirees will have the time to dedicate to that much cardio in addition to the recommended weight training.

	Target zone	% of max HR bpm range	Example duration	Training benefit
Maximize Perfomance	**5** Maximum	90-100% 171-190 bpm	Less than 5 minutes	**Benefits:** Increases maximum sprint race speed **Feels like:** Very exhausting for breathing and muscles **Recommended for:** Very fit persons with athletic training background
	4 Hard	80-90% 152-171 bpm	2-10 minutes	**Benefits:** Increases maximum performance capacity **Feels like:** Muscular fatigue and heavy breathing **Recommended for:** Fit users and for short exercises
Improve Fitness	**3** Moderate	70-80% 133-152 bpm	10-40 minutes	**Benefits:** Improves aerobic fitness **Feels like:** Light muscular fatigue, easy breathing, moderate sweating **Recommended for:** Everybody for typical, moderately long exercises
Lose Weight	**2** Light	60-70% 114-133 bpm	40-80 minutes	**Benefits:** Improves basic endurance and hlps recovery **Feels like:** Comfortable, easy breathing, low muscle load, light sweating **Recommended for:** Everybody for longer and frequently repeated shorter exercises
	1 Very Light	50-60% 104-114 bpm	20-40 minutes	**Benefits:** Improves overall health and metabolism, helps recovery **Feels like:** Very easy for breathing and muscles **Recommended for:** Basic training for novice exercisers, weight management and active recovery

FIGURE 14.1 Training and heart rate zones.

Aim for two or three Zone 2 sessions each week lasting 30 to 60 minutes. But if you only have 20 minutes a couple times a week to devote to Zone 2, that's OK, although I would probably opt for a HIIT workout instead of Zone 2 if the duration is that short.

High-intensity interval training, as the name suggests, is quite intense. It is generally performed in Zones 4 to 5, so your heart rate can get quite high. As such, if you haven't been doing any cardio along with your weight training, I would start with Zone 2 for a couple months to develop a good cardio base before attempting high-intensity intervals.

I recommend one or two interval sessions each week between 20 and 60 minutes of total HIIT workout time. An ideal week for me would be three weight-training sessions, two Zone 2 days, and one HIIT day. And I do throw in those super short rowing intervals (usually 100-meter to 2,000-meter sprints lasting from about 17 seconds up to 9 minutes) on weight-training and non-weight-training days as I feel up to it. These ultrashort HIIT sessions are included in my weekly minute total for HIIT.

However, most of my HIIT sessions use one of three protocols: the Sprint 8, the Norwegian 4 × 4, and 1:2 work-to-rest intervals (e.g. 10 second work, 20 seconds rest for 20 minutes)

Sprint 8: This program involves eight 30-second sprints alternating with 90-second active recovery periods. I use a recumbent bike for these, but you can use any cardio modality you like providing you are pushing your heart into the Zone 4 to 5 range during the sprints (figure 14.2).

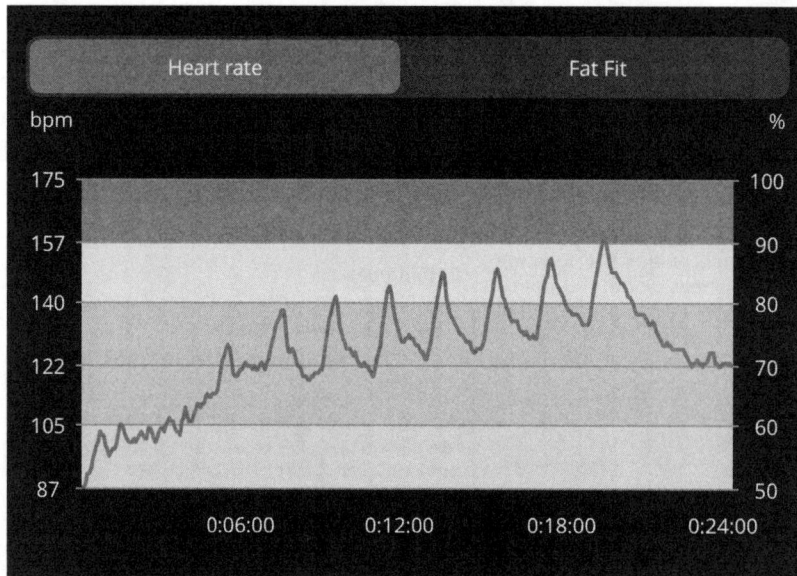

FIGURE 14.2   Sprint 8 training heart rate example.

Norwegian 4 × 4: This protocol uses fewer but longer intervals. Four rounds of four-minute sprints with three-minute recovery periods. Aim to get your heart rate into Zone 4 over the first 90 seconds of the sprint interval and back down into Zone 2 during the recovery periods (figure 14.3).

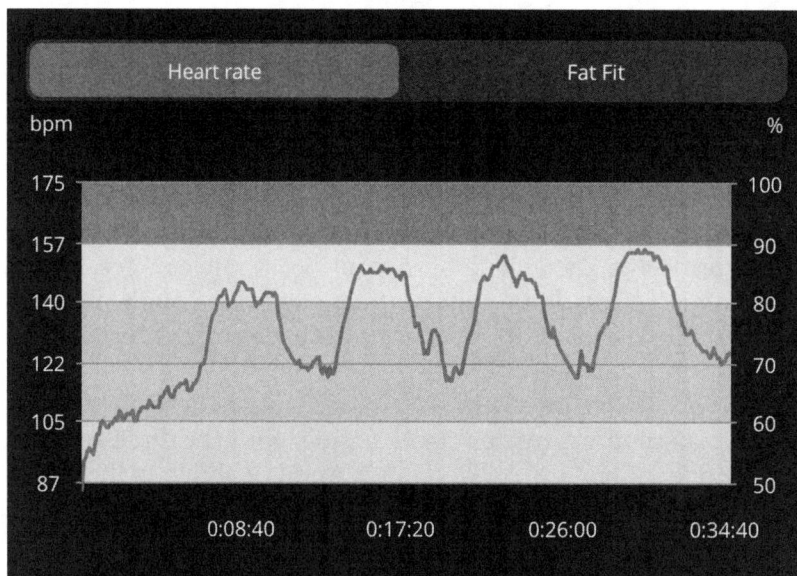

FIGURE 14.3   Norwegian 4 × 4 training heart rate example.

1:2 work-to-rest interval: This method uses a rest period that is twice the length of the work period. I personally like a 10-second sprint with 20 seconds of rest repeated for 20 minutes (40 rounds total; figure 14.4). However, you can do any amount you like, for example, a 15-second sprint with 30 seconds of rest, a 20-second sprint with 40 seconds of rest, and so on.

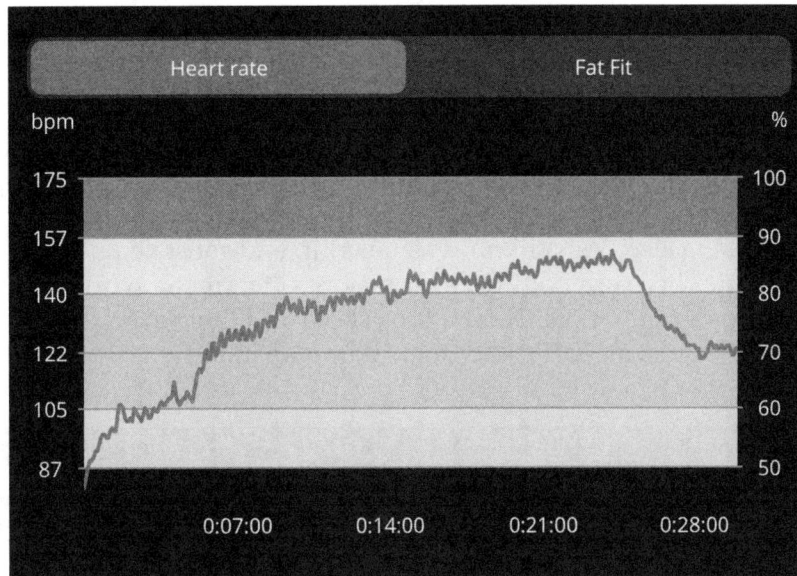

FIGURE 14.4   1:2 work-to-rest interval training heart rate example.

These are my three favorites, but there are countless ways to set up interval training, so feel free to experiment and find something you enjoy and will be consistent with.

Remember, cardio isn't just a side quest—it's part of your core build. It boosts your constitution score, raises your endurance, and keeps your heart strong for the long campaign. After 50, it's not optional. It's the difference between surviving the dungeon or rolling up a new character.

RECOVERY

Let's be real, charging through workouts without sleep or rest isn't hardcore, it's just bad strategy, especially if you're over 50. Recovery isn't a detour from progress; it's the path that makes progress possible. Your energy, strength, and resilience—your real-life hit points—depend on what you do outside the gym as much as inside it. Skimp on sleep, slack on nutrition, and skip rest days, and you'll be setting yourself up to crash before you can conquer anything. Instead, treat recovery like part of your training plan. Prioritize high-quality sleep, fuel up with real food, and build in downtime. Only then will you be ready to take on whatever challenges tomorrow throws your way.

How do you know if you're not recovering properly? Here are a few common indicators (Hospital for Special Surgery 2021):

- **Fatigue and lethargy:** Excessive tiredness, even if you've been sleeping well, is a telltale sign you might be overtraining.

- **Muscle soreness:** This isn't the typical post-workout soreness, but prolonged pain that lasts for days.

- **Decreased performance:** Everyone can have a "coal" day, but if you are consistently weaker in the gym than prior workouts, you likely aren't recovering well. This is another reason a training journal is so valuable.

- **Increased resting heart rate:** Most of us likely have no idea what our resting heart rate is. However, with wearable technology (Apple watch, for example), it can be pretty easy to track. If you find your resting heart rate is higher than normal, you're probably overdoing it.

So what exactly does recovery entail? Well, it's not just sitting on the couch with a bag of chips (as tempting as that might sound). It's about actively supporting your body's natural processes to repair and rebuild stronger.

First, let's talk sleep. We all know we need it, and most of us aren't getting enough! Sleep is when your body does the majority of its repair work, from muscle tissue to hormone regulation. Older adults should aim for seven to nine hours a night (Hirshkowitz et al. 2015), and don't skimp on quality.

Dungeon Master's Guide to Improved Sleep Quality and Hit Point Recovery

- **Cast the lights-out ritual.** Invoke this spell nightly within the same 30-minute window for a bonus on every long-rest recovery roll. Regular sleep timing protects an adventurer's heart and even lowers all-cause mortality (Phillips et al. 2024; Sletten et al. 2023).

- **Don a cloak of shadow and frost.** Enchant your bedchamber to 60 to 67 °F (16–19 °C) and snuff out all wandering light wisps; the chill darkness speeds the journey to deep sleep and recovered hit points (Drerup 2019).

- **Sheathe the screens an hour before bed.** Blue-light dragons from phones, tablets, or e-readers suppress melatonin and nudge your circadian clock later. Stash those artifacts in your bag of holding until morning (Chang et al. 2015).

- **Quaff no potions of perk or ale of haze.** Caffeine taken six hours before bed and alcohol within three hours places a slow-wave hex on your sleep patterns (Drake et al. 2013; Ebrahim et al. 2013).

- **Cast a tranquility spell.** Five minutes of box-breathing or a brief mindfulness session before bed reduces the fight or flight response and improves relaxation and perceived sleep quality (Rusch et al. 2019).

- **Train, then gain.** Weight training warriors should battle the iron during the day or early evening to increase growth hormone release and deep-sleep time, but finish at least two hours before bed or risk a failed sleep-onset saving throw (Stutz et al. 2019).

- **Track and Tweak.** Slip on a ring of restful recall, aka a wearable such as the Oura Ring. These match closely with lab-grade sleep studies for staging your shut-eye, helping you spot trends, and fine-tuning your sleep to recover your hit points (Svensson et al. 2024).

Next on the recovery checklist is nutrition. Nutrition is so important we dedicated all of chapter 3 to it! Make sure you're fueling your body with plenty of protein to support muscle repair, along with a healthy balance of carbohydrates and fats to provide energy and support overall health. Revisit chapter 3 to dial in your optimal nutrition plan.

Hydration is another crucial piece of the recovery puzzle. Water is involved in pretty much every bodily function, so staying hydrated is key to feeling your best, both in and out of the gym. Aim to drink plenty of water throughout the day and consider adding electrolytes if you're sweating buckets during your workouts. Refer to chapter 3 for specific hydration recommendations.

And let's not forget about taking days off from training. Rest days are an essential part of the program, especially as we get older. Your body needs time to recover and rebuild, so don't be afraid to take a day off from the gym every now and then. Use rest days to focus on mobility work, stretching, or simply chilling out and giving your body the break it deserves. Rest days are also great days to get a massage or take a sauna.

Occasionally, you may even need to back off a bit on workout days for a week or two. These are called "deload weeks". You can lighten the weights used, do fewer sets and reps, or even leave out some exercises entirely. Again, I highly recommend a workout journal to keep track of everything and find what works for you.

Finally, don't underestimate the power of stress management and relaxation techniques. Chronic stress can wreak havoc on your body's ability to recover, so make sure you're taking time to unwind and destress on a regular basis. Whether it's through meditation, yoga, or simply taking a leisurely walk in nature, find what works for you and make it a priority.

Remember, recovery isn't just what you do between workouts. It's how you recharge your hit points, refill your mana, and prep for the next mission. And cardio? Skipping cardio is like lowering your constitution score in D&D. It'll weaken you, make you tire more quickly, and leave you less resistant to the attacks from life's dungeons. A little cardio investment keeps your endurance and heart health rolling high. Together, cardio and recovery are the unsung heroes that support your quest for strength. Prioritize sleep, stay hydrated, fuel up like you're building a hero, and give your body the downtime it needs. You're not just training for muscle. You're building resilience, vitality, and longevity. Recovery is your real-life cheat code. Use it.

Since smashing "Start" on page 1, we've side-scrolled through every chapter like heroes in an 8-bit quest. We pumped iron like the *Predator* crew, hacked our macros with MacGyver-level ingenuity, red-lined our cardio like Crockett and Tubbs in a midnight Ferrari, and rolled recovery dice to top off those D&D hit points. Weight training, nutrition, cardio, recovery, we've woven them together into a roadmap Gen Xers can follow to thrive well beyond the half-century mark.

Remember, Gen X, we were the *original* cool kids. Whether you rocked a mullet (guilty!) or teased your bangs to Aqua Net–defying heights, we owned the '80s. Parachute pants, Jordache jeans, Members Only jackets? Check. Walkman clipped to your belt or boombox on your shoulder? Check. And our soundtrack of era-defining rock, rap, and hip-hop anthems still crushes today's playlists. The movies? Don't even get me started; nobody tops our VHS shelf!

We had style, attitude, and grit, traits that never expire. Keep that Beastie Boys–level energy, chase new PRs, and never let anyone tell you you're "too old." Stay strong, stay independent, stay Gen X, and prove once more that the generation raised on MTV still knows how to crank the volume to 11 for life!

REFERENCES

Chapter 1

Bureau of Labor Statistics, U.S. Department of Labor. 2016. "Sports and Exercise Among Americans." *The Economics Daily*. Last modified August 4, 2016. Accessed March 17, 2023. https://www.bls.gov/opub/ted/2016/sports-and-exercise-among-americans.htm.

Cornelissen, Veronique A., and Neil A. Smart. 2013. "Exercise Training for Blood Pressure: A Systematic Review and Meta-Analysis." *Journal of the American Heart Association* 2 (1): e004473. https://doi.org/10.1161/JAHA.112.004473.

Eves, Neil D., and Ronald C. Plotnikoff. 2006. "Resistance Training and Type 2 Diabetes: Considerations for Implementation at the Population Level." *Diabetes Care* 29 (8): 1933-41. https://doi.org/10.2337/dc05-1981.

Friedrich, Cathe. 2023. "5 Medications That Can Hinder Muscle Growth and Exercise Gains." *Cathe Friedrich Blog*. Last modified (approx.) October 2023. Accessed January 18, 2025. https://cathe.com/5-medications-that-can-hinder-muscle-growth-and-exercise-gains.

Healthline. 2018. "These 7 Medications and Workouts Do Not Mix." *Healthline*. Accessed January 18, 2025. https://www.healthline.com/health/medications-workouts-do-not-mix.

Howe, Tracey E., Lynn Rochester, Fiona Neil, Dawn A. Skelton, and Claire Ballinger. 2011. "Exercise for Improving Balance in Older People." *Cochrane Database of Systematic Reviews* 11: CD004963. https://doi.org/10.1002/14651858.CD004963.pub3.

Hurst, Christopher, Stephen M. Robinson, Miles D. Witham, Matthew A. Lamb, Samantha T. Granic, and Avan Aihie Sayer. 2022. "Resistance Exercise as a Treatment for Sarcopenia: Prescription and Delivery." *Age and Ageing* 51 (2): afac003. https://doi.org/10.1093/ageing/afac003.

Iglay, Heidi B., John P. Thyfault, John W. Apolzan, and Wayne W. Campbell. 2007. "Resistance Training and Dietary Protein: Effects on Glucose Tolerance and Contents of Skeletal Muscle Insulin Signaling Proteins in Older Persons." *American Journal of Clinical Nutrition* 85 (4): 1005-1013. https://doi.org/10.1093/ajcn/85.4.1005.

Kruger, Judy, Susan A. Carlson, and David M. Buchner. 2007. "How Active Are Older Americans?" *Preventing Chronic Disease* 4 (3): A53. https://www.ncbi.nlm.nih.gov/pmc/articles/PMC1955422/.

Lansdown, D.A., I. Bendich, D. Motamedi, and B.T. Feeley. 2018. "Imaging-Based Prevalence of Superior Labral Anterior-Posterior Tears Significantly Increases in the Aging Shoulder." *Orthopaedic Journal of Sports Medicine* 6 (9): 2325967118797065. https://doi.org/10.1177/2325967118797065.

Liao, Chun-De, Jau-Yih Tsauo, Yen-Tzu Wu, Cheng-Po Cheng, Hsi-Chung Chen, Yu-Ching Huang, Hao-Chang Chen, and Tain-Hung Liou 2017. "Effects of Protein Supplementation Combined with Resistance Exercise on Body Composition and Physical Function in Older Adults: A Systematic Review and Meta-Analysis." *The American Journal of Clinical Nutrition* 106 (4): 1078-91. https://doi.org/10.3945/ajcn.116.143594.

Liu, C.J., and N.K. Latham. 2009. "Progressive Resistance Strength Training for Improving Physical Function in Older Adults." *Cochrane Database of Systematic Reviews* 3:CD002759.

Lohman, Timothy J., Scott A. Going, Richard Pamenter, Matthew Hall, Thomas Boyden, Linda Houtkooper, Cheryl Ritenbaugh, Lisa Bare, Anabel Hill, and Mikel Aickin. 1995. "Effects of Resistance Training on Regional and Total Bone Mineral Density in Premenopausal Women: A Randomized Prospective Study." *Journal of Bone and Mineral Research* 10 (7): 1015-24. https://doi.org/10.1002/jbmr.5650100705.

Martyn-St James, Marrissa, and Sean Carroll. 2008. "Meta-Analysis of Walking for Preservation of Bone Mineral Density in Postmenopausal Women." *Bone* 43 (3): 521-31. https://doi.org/10.1016/j.bone.2008.05.012.

Pontzer, Herman, Yosuke Yamada, Hiroyuki Sagayama, et al. 2021. "Daily Energy Expenditure Through the Human Life Course." *Science* 373 (6556): 808-12. https://doi.org/10.1126/science.abe5017.

Reid, Kieran F., and Roger A. Fielding. 2012. "Skeletal Muscle Power: A Critical Determinant of Physical Functioning in Older Adults." *Exercise and Sport Sciences Reviews* 40 (1): 4-12. https://doi.org/10.1097/JES.0b013e31823b5f13.

Saleh, Naveed. 2020. "Common Drugs That May Make Exercise Dangerous." MDLinx. Accessed January 18, 2025. https://www.mdlinx.com/article/common-drugs-that-may-make-exercise-dangerous/5GgPmrOXes3prcIp3fDISF.

Sherrington, Catherine, et al. 2019. "Exercise for Preventing Falls in Older People Living in the Community." *Cochrane Database of Systematic Reviews* 2019 (1): CD012424. https://doi.org/10.1002/14651858.CD012424.pub2.

Sohal, Mandeep. 2023. "8 Medications That Can Interfere With Your Workout." *GoodRx Health*. Updated February 6, 2023. Accessed January 18, 2025. https://www.goodrx.com/drugs/side-effects/medications-interfere-with-workout-exercise.

Srikanthan, Preethi, and Arun S. Karlamangla. 2014. "Muscle Mass Index as a Predictor of Longevity in Older Adults." *American Journal of Medicine* 127 (6): 547-53. https://doi.org/10.1016/j.amjmed.2014.02.007. PubMed

Statista. 2023. "Life Expectancy in the United States From 1900 to 2020." Accessed March 16, 2023. https://www.statista.com/statistics/1040079/life-expectancy-united-states-all-time.

Volpi, Elena, Reza Nazemi, and Satoshi Fujita. 2004. "Muscle Tissue Changes With Aging." *Current Opinion in Clinical Nutrition and Metabolic Care* 7 (4): 405-10. https://doi.org/10.1097/01.mco.0000134362.76653.b2.

von Loeffelholz, Christian, and Andreas L. Birkenfeld. 2022. "Non-Exercise Activity Thermogenesis in Human Energy Homeostasis." In Endotext [Internet], edited by Kenneth R. Feingold, Shlomo F. Ahmed, Bryan Anawalt, et al. South Dartmouth, MA: MDText.com, Inc. Updated November 25, 2022. https://www.ncbi.nlm.nih.gov/books/NBK279077/.

Walston, Jeremy D. 2012. "Sarcopenia in Older Adults." *Current Opinion in Rheumatology* 24 (6): 623-27. https://doi.org/10.1097/BOR.0b013e328358d59b.

Westcott, Wayne L. 2012. "Resistance Training Is Medicine: Effects of Strength Training on Health." *Current Sports Medicine Reports* 11 (4): 209-16. https://doi.org/10.1249/JSR.0b013e31825dabb8.

Williams, Mark A., and Kerry J. Stewart. 2009. "Impact of Strength and Resistance Training on Cardiovascular Disease Risk Factors and Outcomes in Older Adults." *Clinics in Geriatric Medicine* 25 (4): 703-14. https://doi.org/10.1016/j.cger.2009.07.003.

Chapter 2

Hutchinson, A. 2016. "Running Preserves 'Motor Units'". *Runner's World*, March 30. https://www.runnersworld.com/health-injuries/a20790871/running-preserves-motor-units/

Hutchinson, Andrew. 2019. "New Report Looks at the Growth of Influencer Marketing on Instagram." *Social Media Today*, December 18, 2019. Accessed January 18, 2025. https://www.socialmediatoday.com/news/new-report-looks-at-the-growth-of-influencer-marketing-on-instagram-1/569277/.

Kovacevic, Ana, Yorgi Mavros, Jennifer J. Heisz, and Maria A. Fiatarone Singh. 2018. "The Effect of Resistance Exercise on Sleep: A Systematic Review of Randomized Controlled Trials." *Sleep Medicine Reviews* 39 (June): 52-68. https://doi.org/10.1016/j.smrv.2017.07.002.

Nuckols, Greg. 2023. "Most Lifters Probably Train Too Light." *Stronger by Science* (Research Spotlight), May 3, 2023. Accessed January 18, 2025. https://www.strongerbyscience.com/research-spotlight-train-light/.

Piasecki, M., A. Ireland, J. Piasecki, et al. 2019. "Long-Term Endurance and Power Training May Facilitate Motor Unit Size Expansion to Compensate for Declining Motor Unit Numbers in Older Age." *Physiologia*, 10.

Zippia. 2023. "Personal Trainer Demographics and Statistics in the US." Accessed January 18, 2025. https://www.zippia.com/personal-trainer-jobs/demographics.

Chapter 3

Åkesson, K., K.-H. William Lau, P. Johnston, E. Imperio, and D.J. Baylink. 1998. "Effects of Short-Term Calcium Depletion and Repletion on Biochemical Marks of Bone Turnover in Young Adult Women." *The Journal of Clinical Endocrinology & Metabolism* 83 (6): 1921-1927. https://doi.org/10.1210/jcem.83.6.4891.

Beshgetoor, D., J.F. Nichols, and I. Rego. 2000. "Effect of Training Mode and Calcium Intake on Bone Mineral Density in Female Master Cyclists, Runners, and Non-Athletes." *International Journal of Sport Nutrition and Exercise Metabolism* 10 (3): 290-301. https://doi.org/10.1123/ijsnem.10.3.290

Burke, L.M., M.L. Ross, L.A. Garvican-Lewis, et al. 2017. "Low Carbohydrate, High Fat Diet Impairs Exercise Economy and Negates the Performance Benefit From Intensified Training in Elite Race Walkers." *The Journal of Physiology* 595 (9): 2785-2807. https://doi.org/10.1113/JP273230

Candow, D.G., P.D. Chilibeck, S.C. Forbes, C.M. Fairman, B. Gualano, and H. Roschel (2022). "Creatine Supplementation for Older Adults: Focus on Sarcopenia, Osteoporosis, Frailty and Cachexia." *Bone* 162: 116467. https://doi.org/10.1016/j.bone.2022.116467

Devarshi, P.P., K. Gustafson, R.W. Grant, and S.H. Mitmesser. 2023. "Higher Intake of Certain Nutrients Among Older Adults Is Associated With Better Cognitive Function: An Analysis of NHANES 2011-2014." *BMC Nutrition* 9 (1). https://doi.org/10.1186/s40795-023-00802-0

Domínguez, R., E. Cuenca, J. Maté-Muñoz, et al. 2017. "Effects of Beetroot Juice Supplementation on Cardiorespiratory Endurance in Athletes. A Systematic Review." *Nutrients* 9 (1): 43. www.ncbi.nlm.nih.gov/pmc/articles/PMC5295087/

Fogelholm, M., H. Sievänen, A. Heinonen, et al. 1997. "Association Between Weight Cycling History and Bone Mineral Density in Premenopausal Women." *Osteoporosis International* 7 (4): 354-358. https://doi.org/10.1007/Bf01623777

Heileson, J.L., S.B. Machek, D.R. Harris, et al. 2023. "The Effect of Fish Oil Supplementation on Resistance Training-Induced Adaptations." *Journal of the International Society of Sports Nutrition* 20 (1). https://doi.org/10.1080/15502783.2023.2174704

Janssen, I., S.B. Heymsfield, Z. Wang, and R. Ross. 2000. "Skeletal Muscle Mass and Distribution in 468 Men and Women Aged 18-88 Yr." *Journal of Applied Physiology* 89 (1): 81-88. https://doi.org/10.1152/jappl.2000.89.1.81

Kerstetter, J.E., K.O. O'Brien, and K.L. Insogna. 2003. "Dietary Protein, Calcium Metabolism, and Skeletal Homeostasis Revisited." *The American Journal of Clinical Nutrition* 78 (3): 584S592S. https://doi.org/10.1093/ajcn/78.3.584s

Louis, J., F. Vercruyssen, O. Dupuy, and T. Bernard. 2019. "Nutrition for Master Athletes: Is There a Need for Specific Recommendations?" *Journal of Aging and Physical Activity* 28 (3): 1-10. https://doi.org/10.1123/japa.2019-0190

Tang, J.E., D.R. Moore, G.W. Kujbida, M.A. Tarnopolsky, and S.M. Phillips. 2009. "Ingestion of Whey Hydrolysate, Casein, or Soy Protein Isolate: Effects on Mixed Muscle Protein Synthesis at Rest and Following Resistance Exercise in Young Men." *Journal of Applied Physiology* 107 (3): 987-992. https://doi.org/10.1152/japplphysiol.00076.2009

Tarnopolsky, M., A. Zimmer, J. Paikin, et al. 2007. "Creatine Monohydrate and Conjugated Linoleic Acid Improve Strength and Body Composition Following Resistance Exercise in Older Adults." *PLoS ONE* 2 (10): e991. https://doi.org/10.1371/journal.pone.0000991

Tzankoff, S.P., and A.H. Norris. 1977. "Effect of Muscle Mass Decrease on Age-Related BMR Changes." *Journal of Applied Physiology* 43 (6): 1001-1006.

Wax, B., C.M. Kerksick, A.R. Jagim, J.J. Mayo, B.C. Lyons, and R.B. Kreider. 2021. "Creatine for Exercise and Sports Performance, With Recovery Considerations for Healthy Populations." *Nutrients* 13 (6): 1915. https://doi.org/10.3390/nu13061915

Chapter 5

Bishop, David. 2003. "Warm-Up I: Potential Mechanisms and the Effects of Passive Warm-Up on Exercise Performance." *Sports Medicine* 33 (6): 439-54. https://doi.org/10.2165/00007256-200333060-00005.

Fradkin, Andrea J., Tsharni T. Zazryn, and James M. Smoliga. 2010. "Effects of Warming-Up on Physical Performance: A Systematic Review With Meta-Analysis." *Journal of Strength and Conditioning Research* 24 (1): 140-48. https://doi.org/10.1519/JSC.0b013e3181c643a0.

McGowan, Courtney J., David B. Pyne, Kevin G. Thompson, and Ben Rattray. 2015. "Warm-Up Strategies for Sport and Exercise: Mechanisms and Applications." *Sports Medicine* 45 (11): 1523-46. https://doi.org/10.1007/s40279-015-0376-x.

Shellock, Frederic G., and William E. Prentice. 1985. "Warming-Up and Stretching for Improved Physical Performance and Prevention of Sports-Related Injuries." *Sports Medicine* 2 (4): 267-78. https://doi.org/10.2165/00007256-198502040-00004.

Stewart, Iain B., and Michael G. Sleivert. 1998. "The Effect of Warm-Up Intensity on Range of Motion and Anaerobic Performance." *Journal of Orthopaedic and Sports Physical Therapy* 27 (2): 154-61. https://doi.org/10.2519/jospt.1998.27.2.154.

Chapter 7

Celis-Morales, Carlos A., Paul Welsh, Donald M. Lyall, et al. 2018. "Associations of Grip Strength With Cardiovascular, Respiratory, and Cancer Outcomes and All-Cause Mortality: Prospective Cohort Study of Half a Million UK Biobank Participants." *BMJ* 361: k1651. https://doi.org/10.1136/bmj.k1651.

Cooper, R., D. Kuh, and R. Hardy. 2010. "Objectively Measured Physical Capability Levels and Mortality: Systematic Review and Meta-Analysis." *BMJ* 341: c4467. https://doi.org/10.1136/bmj.c4467

Leong, D.P., K. Teo, S. Rangarajan, et al. 2015. "Prognostic Value of Grip Strength: Findings from the Prospective Urban Rural Epidemiology (PURE) Study." *The Lancet* 386 (9990): 266-73. https://doi.org/10.1016/S0140-6736(14)62000-6

Chapter 9

Newman, A., Kupelian, V., Visser, E., Simonsick, B., Goodpaster, S., et al. 2006. "Strength, but Not Muscle Mass, Is Associated with Mortality in the Health, Aging and Body Composition Study Cohort." *Journal of Gerontology*: Series A61 (1): 72–77. https://doi.org/10.1093/gerona/61.1.72.

Ortega, F., Silventoinen, K., Tynelius, P., and Rasmussen, F. 2012. "Muscular Strength in Male Adolescents and Premature Death: Cohort Study of One Million Participants." *BMJ* 345: e7279. https://doi.org/10.1136/bmj.e7279.

Chapter 10

Schoenfeld, Brad J., Daniel I. Ogborn, and James W. Krieger. 2015. "Effect of Repetition Duration During Resistance Training on Muscle Hypertrophy: A Systematic Review and Meta-Analysis." *Sports Medicine* 45 (4): 577-85. https://doi.org/10.1007/s40279-015-0304-0.

Schoenfeld, Brad J., Zachary K. Pope, Frank M. Benik, et al. 2016. "Longer Interset Rest Periods Enhance Muscle Strength and Hypertrophy in Resistance-Trained Men." *Journal of Strength and Conditioning Research* 30 (7): 1805-12. https://doi.org/10.1519/JSC.0000000000001272.

Chapter 14

American Heart Association. 2023. "American Heart Association Recommendations for Physical Activity in Adults and Kids." Last reviewed January 12, 2023. Accessed February 12, 2025. https://www.heart.org/en/healthy-living/fitness/fitness-basics/aha-recs-for-physical-activity-in-adults.

Chang, Anne-Marie, Daniel Aeschbach, Jeanne F. Duffy, and Charles A. Czeisler. 2015. "Evening Use of Light-Emitting eReaders Negatively Affects Sleep, Circadian Timing, and Next-Morning Alertness." *Proceedings of the National Academy of Sciences* 112 (4): 1232-37. https://doi.org/10.1073/pnas.1418490112.

Drake, Christopher L., Timothy Roehrs, James Shambroom, and Thomas Roth. 2013. "Caffeine Effects on Sleep Taken 0, 3, or 6 Hours Before Going to Bed." *Journal of Clinical Sleep Medicine* 9 (11): 1195-1200. https://doi.org/10.5664/jcsm.3170.

Drerup, Michelle. 2019. "What's the Best Temperature for Sleep?" *Cleveland Clinic Health Essentials*, July 16, 2019. https://health.clevelandclinic.org/what-is-the-ideal-sleeping-temperature-for-my-bedroom (accessed June 1, 2025).

Ebrahim, Irshaad O., Colin M. Shapiro, Adrian J. Williams, and Peter B. Fenwick. 2013. "Alcohol and Sleep I: Effects on Normal Sleep." *Alcoholism: Clinical and Experimental Research* 37 (4): 539-49. https://doi.org/10.1111/acer.12006.

Hirshkowitz, M., K. Whiton, S.M. Albert, et al. 2015. "National Sleep Foundation's Sleep Time Duration Recommendations: Methodology and Results Summary." *Sleep Health* 1 (1): 40-43. https://doi.org/10.1016/j.sleh.2014.12.010

Hospital for Special Surgery. 2021. "Overtraining: Signs and Solutions." Accessed February 12, 2025. https://www.hss.edu/health-library/move-better/overtraining.

Kokkinos, P., Faselis, C., Samuel, B., Pittaras, A., Doumas, M., et al. 2022. "Cardiorespiratory Fitness and Mortality Risk Across the Spectra of Age, Race, and Sex." *Journal of the American College of Cardiology* 80 (6): 598–609. https://doi.org/10.1016/j.jacc.2022.05.031.

Kraemer, W.J., and N.A. Ratamess. 2004. "Fundamentals of Resistance Training: Progression and Exercise Prescription." *Medicine and Science in Sports and Exercise* 36 (4): 674-688. https://doi.org/10.1249/01.mss.0000121945.36635.61

Mandolesi, L., A. Polverino, S. Montuori, et al. 2018. "Effects of Physical Exercise on Cognitive Functioning and Wellbeing: Biological and Psychological Benefits." *Frontiers in Psychology* 9: 509. https://doi.org/10.3389/fpsyg.2018.00509

Mandsager, K., Harb, S. Cremer, P., Phelan, D., Nissen, S., Jaber, J. 2018. "Association of Cardiorespiratory Fitness with Long-Term Mortality among Adults Undergoing Exercise Treadmill Testing." *JAMA Network Open* 1 (6): e183605. https://doi.org/10.1001/jamanetworkopen.2018.3605.

Oja, P., S. Titze, A. Bauman, et al. 2011. "Health Benefits of Cycling: A Systematic Review." *Scandinavian Journal of Medicine and Science in Sports* 21 (4): 496-509. https://doi.org/10.1111/j.1600-0838.2011.01280.x

Phillips, Andrew J. K., Daniel P. Windred, Cuilin Gao, et al. 2024. "Sleep Regularity Is a Stronger Predictor of Mortality Risk Than Sleep Duration." *Sleep* 47 (1): zsad253. https://doi.org/10.1093/sleep/zsad253.

Rusch, Heather L., Michael Rosario, Lisa M. Levison, Anlys Olivera, Whitney S. Livingston, Tianxia Wu, and Jessica M. Gill. 2019. "The Effect of Mindfulness Meditation on Sleep Quality: A Systematic Review and Meta-Analysis of Randomized Controlled Trials." *Annals of the New York Academy of Sciences* 1445 (1): 5-16. https://doi.org/10.1111/nyas.13996.

Sletten, Tracey L., Matthew D. Weaver, Russell G. Foster, David Gozal, Elizabeth B. Klerman, Shantha M. W. Rajaratnam, et al. 2023. "The Importance of Sleep Regularity: A Consensus Statement of the National Sleep Foundation Sleep Timing and Variability Panel." *Sleep Health* 9 (6): 801-20. https://doi.org/10.1016/j.sleh.2023.07.016.

Stutz, Janine, Remo Eiholzer, and Christina M. Spengler. 2019. "Effects of Evening Exercise on Sleep in Healthy Participants: A Systematic Review and Meta-Analysis." *Sports Medicine* 49 (2): 269-87. https://doi.org/10.1007/s40279-018-1015-0.

Svensson, Thomas, Riikka Puuronen, Markku Partinen, et al. 2024. "Validity and Reliability of the Oura Ring Generation 3 With the Oura Sleep Staging Algorithm 2.0 When Compared to Multi-Night Ambulatory Polysomnography." *Sleep Medicine* 106: 123-31. https://doi.org/10.1016/j.sleep.2024.01.020.

Willis, L.H., C.A. Slentz, L.A. Bateman, et al. 2012. "Effects of Aerobic and/or Resistance Training on Body Mass and Fat Mass in Overweight or Obese Adults." *Journal of Applied Physiology* 113 (12): 1831-1837. https://doi.org/10.1152/japplphysiol.01370.2011

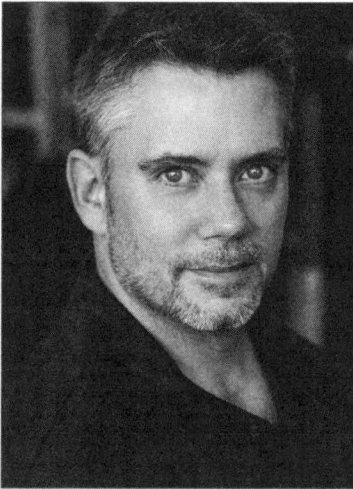

Chad Landers is a 1991 graduate of the University of Illinois Urbana-Champaign with a bachelor's degree in kinesiology. He has a graduate diploma in sports nutrition from the International Olympic Committee (IOC) and he was the National Strength and Conditioning Association (NSCA) Personal Trainer of the Year in 2018.

Landers is in his 32nd year as a personal trainer in Los Angeles, California, and has owned and operated PUSH Private Fitness, a personal training–only gym, for over 20 years. He is known for his work with actors and musicians who need to look their best for the stage and screen. Current and former clients include William (Billy) Zabka, Duff McKagan, Sarah Hyland, Robbie Amell, Lyndsy Fonseca, and Corbin Bleu, among others.

In addition to competing in the sport of powerlifting, Landers enjoys writing and public speaking. He has been featured in *Men's Health*, *Women's Health*, *People*, *AARP The Magazine*, Onnit, Yahoo!, Personal Fitness Professional, and Personal Trainer Development Center and has been a guest on numerous podcasts.

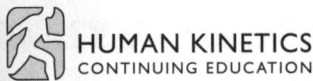

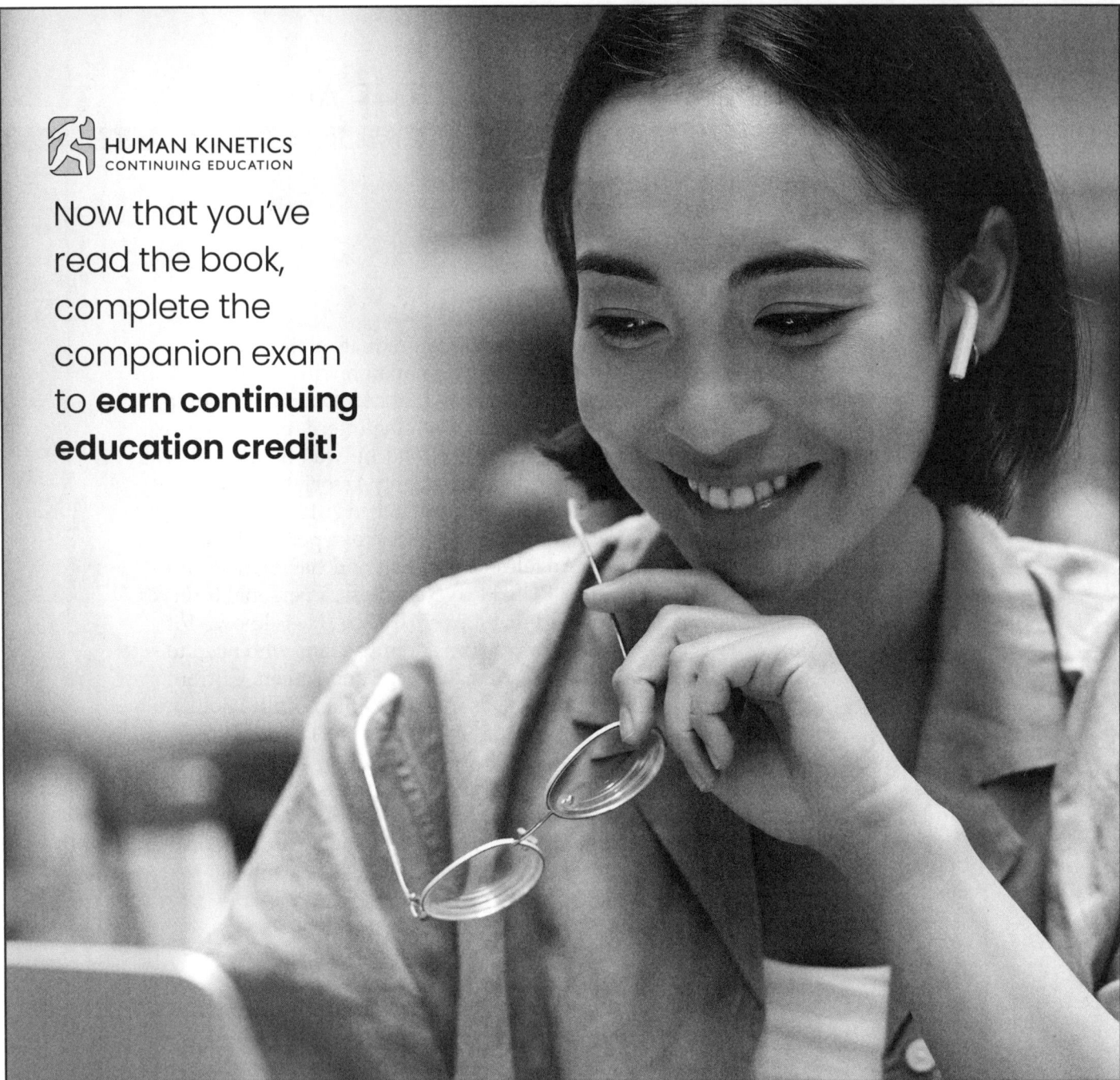

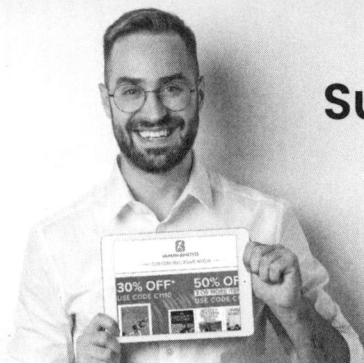